EMERGENCY AND INTENSIVE CARE MEDICINE

THE CONUNDRUM OF TOXIC EPIDERMAL NECROLYSIS

EMERGENCY AND INTENSIVE CARE MEDICINE

Additional books in this series can be found on Nova's website under the Series tab.

Additional e-books in this series can be found on Nova's website under the e-book tab.

EMERGENCY AND INTENSIVE CARE MEDICINE

THE CONUNDRUM OF TOXIC EPIDERMAL NECROLYSIS

GÉRALD E. PIÉRARD
PHILIPPE PAQUET
SERGE JENNES
CLAUDINE FRANCHIMONT

NOVA BIOMEDICAL

New York

Additional color graphics may be available in the e-book version of this book.

Library of Congress Cataloging-in-Publication Data

ISBN: 978-1-63482-068-4
Library of Congress Control Number: 2015930886

Published by Nova Science Publishers, Inc. † New York

Contents

Preface

It has long been recognized that skin is a vital organ to life because it offers a semi-permeable barrier between the homeostatic internal milieu and its hostile environmental outside. Therefore, any severe and widespread alteration of the skin represents a potential life-threatening condition. Such a skin deficiency is occasionally induced by adverse drug reactions (ADR). In this context, drug-induced toxic epidermal necrolysis (TEN) represents the archetype of a set of severe conditions somewhat similar to extensive thermal and chemical burns.

Aided by recent vast advances in technology, ADR research including TEN has surged forward, and publications have mushroomed. However, TEN remains occasionally a puzzling condition for both the clinician at the bedside and in the laboratory. This monograph is fully updated with particular emphasis on clinico-pathologic correlations and recent treatment concepts. It is in line with considerable progress gained during the two past decades. The extension and deepening of our knowledge of TEN is evident at all levels, from the purely morphologic to the molecular and functional aspects. The scope of the monograph includes biologic aspects, clinico-pathologic characteristics, and therapeutic advances. A series of important questions are reviewed and discussed in order to cross-fertilize ideas and advances in different fields of biomedical sciences.

Skin ADR are frequent, and their pathomechanisms are varied. Wherever the clinician exercises a high degree of ADR suspicion, the patient is probably spared discomfort and ailments related to a large variety of disease manifestations. Indeed, most skin ADR are commonly recognized by individual experience, but the link with a specific drug derives from the collective experience of published evidence. TEN is a rare condition and represents the most severe ADR corresponding to a "disease of medical progress". In whatever way, we are still waiting for advanced progress in our understanding of cutaneous ADR. Indeed, a clear identification of the various clinical forms is a prerequisite for elucidating their specific pharmacologic and immunologic mechanisms. The TEN pathways remain in part uncovered. However, major advances were reached in recent years at the two ends of the TEN pathobiology. They deal with: (a) altered metabolic pathways of drugs in some patients leading to reactive toxic metabolites, (b) an improved understanding of the diverse immune cell implications, and (c) new therapeutic attempts.

Of note, eye alterations in TEN are of the utmost importance and need to be adequately and immediately managed. The only hope of influencing prognosis is the modulation of the ocular disease process during its acute stage. TEN patients should be urgently examined by an ophthalmologist upon hospital admission. It is crucial that the consulting ophthalmologists be knowledgeable in the proper evaluation and management of TEN. The application of specialized treatments in severe ocular damages essentially prevents the chronic phase from occurring consequently allowing patients to avoid lifelong ocular pain, visual disability and the need for some costly and difficult treatments that are only partially effective.

Written primarily for physicians keen in dermatology and ophthalmology practice, whether neophytes, seasoned veterans, or researchers, this monograph should be useful to any scientist interested in biomedical disciplines. The emphasis of the present TEN monograph is to fill some gaps between standard textbooks of dermatology and medicine, and to cover the current experience of managing actual patients, the ongoing search about ADR pathobiology, and recent trends in therapeutic developments. This monograph is intended for medical students, dermatologists, ophthalmologists, researchers, primary-care and intensive care physicians, the medical staff taking care of inpatient and outpatient clinics including burn units, and persons in charge of drug companies.

We sincerely hope that this booklet will provide valuable advice to the readers, and that it will stimulate new advances in the identification and treatment of cutaneous ADR. Our intention is far from deliberately discouraging the young explorer from venturing into new medical territories, whether for the sheer love of learning or for more practical reasons. Clearly, the scientific adventurer should proceed only if the researcher is equipped, with an idea and the basic knowledge, a wealth of keen senses, an absence of bias, and a spontaneous readiness to accept facts.

Where this monograph appears incomplete, it is because our knowledge of TEN is still limited and fragmented. If it contains some errors, it is because some of the available facts, in the morphologic or molecular ground, are not yet fully or exactly known. The dizzying pace of dermatology, ophthalmology, dermatopathology, and molecular biology is like a tide providing powerful methods available as a matter of routine for practitioners facing towards TEN. Just believing what one sees is occasionally a snare and a delusion. The skin does not give up all its secrets at a glance. Scrutinizing in depth skin biology is much more accurate and stimulates curiosity. It marshals the observe ingenuities to see beyond the first glance.

We would like to convey our deep appreciation to all over colleagues who offered their stimulating and outstanding cooperation in the conception of the prevent booklet. In a very real sense, this monograph is the product of a team effort. In support to the four authors listed on the case, we acknowledge the contributions over the recent years of W. Al Saleh, J.E. Arrese, C. Courtin, P. Damas, D. De Groote, P. Delvenne, R. Greimers, T. Hermanns-Lê, P. Humbert, E. Jacob, S. Kaveri, M. Lesuisse, G. Mazzuchelli, M.A. Meuwis, A.F. Nikkels, B.V. Nusgens, J. Pirson, P. Quatresooz, M.A. Reginster, C. Ribbens, A.F. Rousseau and N. Schaaf-Lafontaine.

Our indebtedness does not end there. Our heartfelt appreciation and special thanks go to Mrs. Ida Leclercq for her skilful secretarial assistance. She organized, supervised, checked for accuracy, and devoted herself unstintingly to every detail of the book.

Gérald E. Piérard, MD, PhD
Guest Professor, LABIC Laboratory
Department of Clinical Sciences
Liège University, BE-4000 Liège, Belgium
Honoray Professor,
University of Franche-Comté,
F-25000 Besançon, France
E-mail: gerald.pierard@ulg.ac.be

Philippe Paquet, MD, PhD
Department of Dermatopathology, Unilab Lg
CHU Sart Tilman, BE-4000 Liège, Belgium
E-mail: p.paquet@chu.ulg.ac.be

Serge Jennes, MD
Burn Unit
Queen Astrid Military Hospital,
BE-1120 Neder-over-Heembeek, Belgium
E-mail: serge.jennes@mil.be

Claudine Franchimont, MD, PhD
Department of Dermatopathology, Unilab Lg
CHU Sart Tilman, BE-4000 Liège, Belgium
E-mail: claudine.franchimont@ulg.ac.be

Introduction

By and large, the ADR spectrum exhibits a variety of clinical and biological presentations. The resulting diseases frequently affect the skin, in particular the group of severe cutaneous adverse reactions (SCAR). Among them, drug-induced TEN, formerly known under its eponym Lyell's syndrome [1], is a potential dreadful life-threatening condition. It currently corresponds to one of the most dramatic dermatological emergencies. It is basically characterized by a sudden extensive destruction of the epidermis and a diversity of mucosal epithelia. It affects people of both genders, at all ages, and of any ethnic background. The yearly incidence of TEN reaches about 1-3/10^6 individuals in Western populations [2-6]. The 25-40% TEN mortality rate mainly results from a set of secondary metabolic failures primarily affecting the lungs and kidneys, and from microbial septicemia following loss of epithelial integrity [7-9]. The risk is even higher in elderly patients, and in presence of large surface area of epidermal destruction. Potential offending microorganisms are varied including bacteria (mainly *Staphylococcus* spp and *Pseudomonas aeruginosa*) [10], and more rarely some fungi (*Candida albicans, Mucor* spp, ...) [11, 12]. The pathogenesis of TEN is not fully understood, but several relevant observations report that any proposed mechanism must accommodate to the constant epithelial destruction. Recent findings about ADR pathogenesis in general are probably highly relevant [13-23]. The TEN pathobiology, the clinical aspects, the differential diagnoses and the sequels are thoroughly reviewed in this monograph.

General practitioners are potentially at the front line for early diagnosis of most ADR. In addition, several specialized medical disciplines are directly involved in the management of TEN patients. Due to the major implication of cutaneous and mucosal epithelia, dermatologists represent a key group. In addition, ophthalmologists are particularly concerned about the specific taking care of the eye damages. The global management of the patients requires emergency and intensive care hospitalization in a burn unit where adequate systemic survival management, local care of large skin surface necrosis and germ-preserved environment are guaranteed. Other medical disciplines including infectiologists are occasionally concerned by TEN patients.

Scholars of the skin, regardless of their training, will find a great deal of interesting material in this monograph. For experimental dermatologists, this volume is a must. Now, to work!

Acronyms and Abbreviations

ACSR	Antifolate cytotoxic skin reaction
ADR	Adverse drug reaction
AGEP	Acute generalized exanthematous pustulosis
AIDS	Acquired immunodeficiency syndrome
AM	Amniotic membrane
ARDS	Acute respiratory distress syndrome
ATP	Adenosine triphosphate
BFDR	Bullous fixed drug reaction
BrdU	Bromodeoxyuridine
Ca^{2+}	Calcium
CK	Cytokeratin
CLA	Cutaneous lymphocytes antigen
CP450	Cytochrome P450
CSA	Cyclosporine A
CTL	Cytotoxic T lymphocyte
Cyt C	Cytochrome C
DD	Dermal dendrocyte
DISC	Death-inducing signaling complex
DNA	Desoxyribonucleic acid
DR	Death receptor
DRL	Death receptor ligand
DRESS	Drug rash with eosinophilia and systemic symptoms
EM	Erythema multiforme
EMU	Epidermal melanin unit
ESC	Epidermal stem cell
FADD	Fas-associated death domain
Fas	CD95

FasL	Fas ligand
FasR	Fas receptor
FDE	Fixed drug eruption
FMM	Faint mosaic melanoderma
GMS	Gomori methenamine silver
GSH	Glutathione
GST	Glutathione-S-transferase
GVHR	Graft-versus-host reaction
HFP	Hair follicle privilege
HIV	Human immunodeficiency virus
HLA	Human leucocyte antigen
HSV	Herpes simplex virus
^{3}H-TdR	Tritiated thymidine
IAS	Illness auxiliary score
ICAM-1	Intercellular adhesion molecule 1
IFN	Interferon
IL	Interleukin
iNOS	Inducible NO synthase
IVIg	Intravenous immunoglobulin
LFA-1	Lymphocytes function-associated antigen-1
mFasL	Membrane-bound Fas ligand
MHC	Major histocompatibility complex
MMP	Matrix metalloproteinase
MOMP	Mitochondrial outer-membrane permeabilization
MTX	Methotrexate
NAC	N-acetylcysteine
NFkB	Nuclear factor kappa B
NK	Natural killer (CD56)
NO	Nitric oxide
PAS	Periodic acid-Schiff
PEU	Proliferative epidermal unit
PK	Protein kinase
PMC	Post-mitotic cell
PTTB	Partial thickness thermal burn
PTX	Pemetrexed
RCM	Reflectance confocal microscopy
RNA	Ribonucleic acid
ROS	Reactive oxygen species
SCAR	Severe cutaneous adverse reaction

SCD	Stem cell deficiency
SCM	Skin capacitance mapping
SCORTEN	TEN-specific severity of illness score
SCV	Skin color volume
SERCA	Sarco-endodplasmic reticulum Ca^{2+} - ATP
sFasL	Soluble FasL
SJS	Stevens-Johnson syndrome
SSSS	Staphylococcal scalded skin syndrome
sTNF	Soluble TNF
sTNF-R	Soluble TNF receptor
TAC	Transitory amplifier cell
TBSA	Total body surface area
TCR	T cell receptor
TEN	Toxic epidermal necrolysis
TGF	Tumor growth factor
TNF	Tumor necrosis factor
TNF-R1	TNF receptor 1
TRAIL	TNF-related apoptosis-inducing ligand
UVL	Ultraviolet light
VAS	Visual-analog scale

Part I: General Considerations

Chapter 1

From Lyell's Syndrome to Toxic Epidermal Necrolysis

The seminal report about some previously unidentified dramatic skin scalding disorders was published about 60 years ago [1]. Initially, they were named toxic epidermal necrolysis, but its eponym "Lyell's syndrome" prevailed in the literature. At that time, the heterogeneity in both the clinical presentations and outcomes, as well as their distinct origins were progressively disclosed. In some cases, the causative involvement of Staphylococcus aureus spp. was pointed out. This latter condition is currently identified as the staphylococcal scalded skin syndrome (SSSS). Other cases of the Lyell's syndrome appeared as the consequence of drug-induced conditions presently identified under two distinct conditions named TEN or generalized fixed drug eruption (FDE). The TEN concept as a potential life-threatening dermatologic disease was progressively refined [2].

A number of drugs have been reported to induce a variety of skin eruptions, ranging from mild maculopapular exanthema to potential life-threatening conditions [24, 25]. For years, the definitions and nomenclature of cutaneous ADR remained confusing, and various synonyms and eponyms were offered to describe them. Nowadays, ADR are recognized to cause more than 80% of TEN cases [26]. Some specific infections, such as Herpes simplex virus (HSV)-6 and Mycoplasma pneumoniae, have been occasionally involved in a few TEN cases [27, 28]. Such causal relationships are not topical in most research projects.

TEN is characterized by epidermal necrosis extending over 30% of the total body surface area (TBSA). Tissue sloughing off commonly runs for 10-

20 days after discontinuation of the offending drug. When skin detachment remains limited to less than 10% TBSA, the condition is referred to as the Stevens-Johnson syndrome (SJS). When sloughing involves 10 to 30% of TBSA, it is referred to as SJS/TEN overlap [3-6].

In addition to the epidermal destruction, TEN alters a series of other specific organs covered by a pluristratified squamous epithelium, particularly the oral cavity and the eyeball, as well as the esophagus, bronchial airways and vagina. Severe other complications and secondary multisystemic involvements are commonly encountered in TEN. Intestinal and renal lesions, acute pancreatitis and hematologic disturbances (lymphopenia, anemia, disseminated intravascular coagulation) are possible. Metabolic failures of internal organs probably follow and result from the primary destruction of large areas of stratified epithelia, leading to seemingly cytokine storms.

Several groups of patients are at higher risk for developing TEN, such as bone marrow transplant recipients, patients with systemic lupus erythematosus, and patients infected with the human immunodeficiency virus (HIV), including those with the acquired immunodeficiency syndrome (AIDS). A number of TEN cases have been reported in these patients reflecting either extended exposures to drugs or a higher risk of reaction than for other consumers of the same drugs. The yearly incidence of TEN among AIDS patients has been estimated at about 1 to 1,000 compared to 1-3 to million in the general population.

At present, the vast majority of TEN cases are apparently caused by an idiosyncratic ADR. The various presumed pathogenic mechanisms remain conflicting, and the evidence for the benefits of many individual treatments remains poor [29]. Arguments from evidence-based medicine are lacking in absence of controlled studies involving large numbers of patients. This condition is quite impossible to meet due to the rarity of TEN.

Chapter 2

The Keratinocyte, Major Target and Actor

TEN specific pathomechanisms apparently involve only multistratified epithelia, keratinized or not. The epidermis is a stratified keratinized epithelium. Multistratified non-keratinized epithelia are present in the mouth, esophagus, vagina, anal canal, vestibule of the nasal cavity, larynx, conjunctiva, cornea and oropharynx. Both, the trachea and the bronchial tree are lined by a pseudostratified epithelium. They are commonly involved in the TEN initial phases. This could be due to metaplasia. Indeed, under certain physiologic or pathologic conditions, some epithelial tissues undergo a series of transformations into another epithelial type.

In areas exposed to direct airflow like trachea and bronchi, a transformation from typical pseudostratified epithelium to stratified squamous epithelium is common since it provides more protection from attrition than the regular respiratory epithelium. This is particularly evident for smokers, in whom the increased particulate and gaseous pollutants induce such changes in the cell organization of the respiratory tree.

The relationship between TEN pathomechanisms and the primary specific involvement of multistratified epithelia remain to be established. Keratinocytes represent the central initial cells systematically destroyed in the TEN epidermis (Figure 1). The lesions resemble the effects of boric acid ingestion [30]. A series of features support a complex pathogenic mechanism underlying TEN [6, 9].

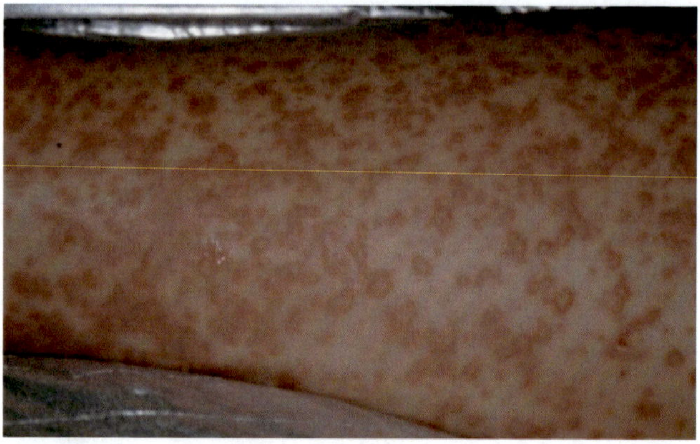

a

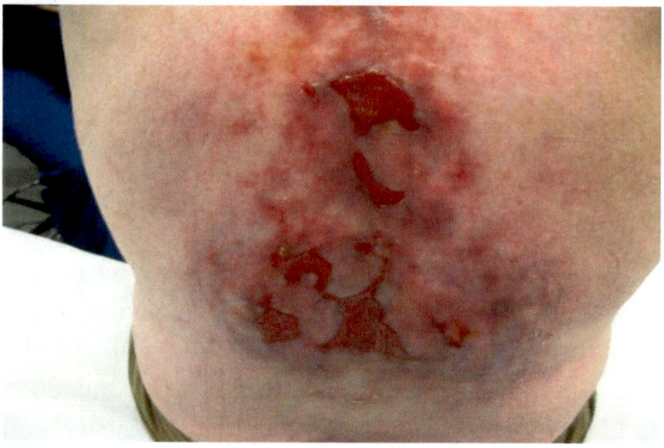

b

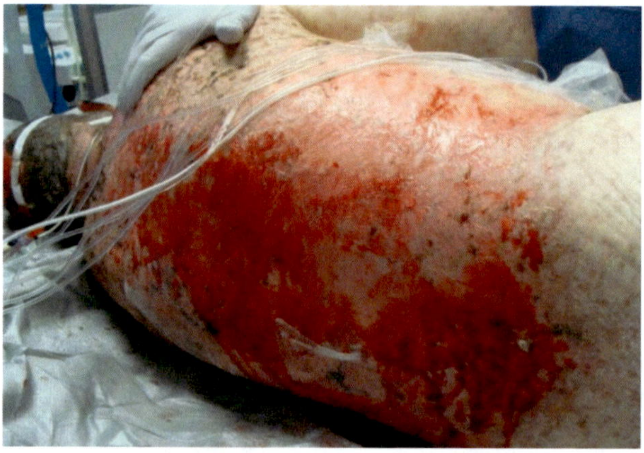

c

Figure 1. (Continued).

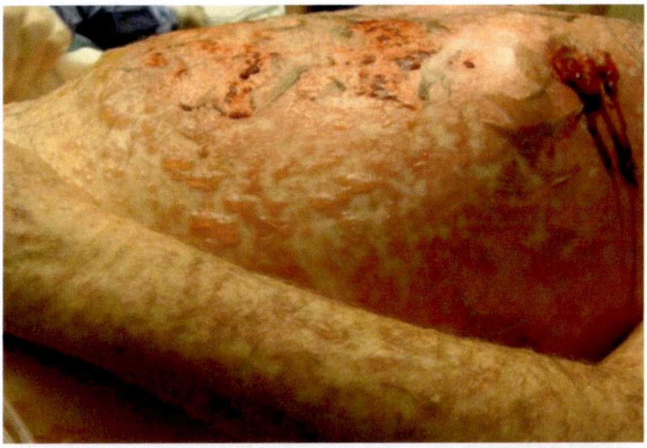

d

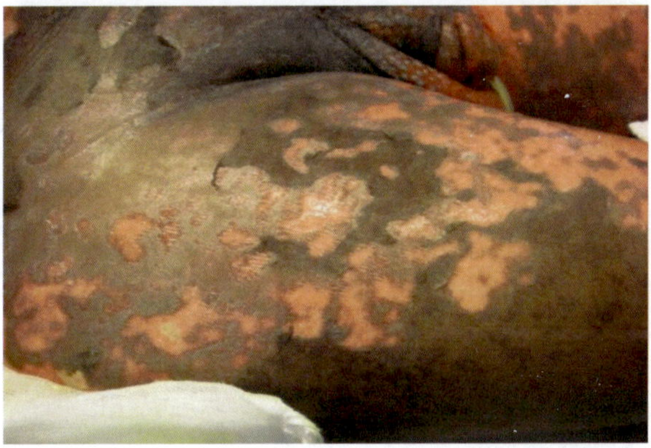

e

Figure 1. Bright red macules in the TEN extension phase: a - widespread dispersion of lesions. b - dermo-epidermal sloughing off with erosions. c - widespread epidermal sloughing off. d - diffuse epidermal alterations.

The epithelium plays an important role in detoxification of certain chemicals and drugs. Such a process is roughly similar by some aspects to the liver function. Keratinocytes exert a prominent bioactivation activity of drugs through various transport-associated and detoxifying enzymes [31].

Some drug metabolites generated by the cytochrome P450 (CP450) system exert toxic effects on epithelial cells when they are not rapidly detoxified. The constitutive presence of CP450 3A, and the potential induction of CP450 1A are documented in the human epidermis [32]. Some molecular investigations ascribe a major role for flavin-containing mono-oxygenase-3 and other peroxidases in the bioactivation of sulfonamides in human keratinocytes [33]. In addition, N-acetyltransferase-1 activity present in healthy keratinocytes is apparently decreased in TEN skin [34] and mucosae (Figure 2). Such a lowered activity potentially decreases the skin clearance of the offending drug, allowing more drug to be metabolized through oxidative pathways [6].

Most TEN lesions contain only a scanty inflammatory cell infiltrate [9]. Of note, the liver is globally preserved in TEN, or only moderately impacted compared to the major epidermal involvement. Therefore, it is likely that the presumed offending drug metabolites do not originate from the liver, but rather the adverse drug bioactivation is primarily keratinocyte-driven [31].

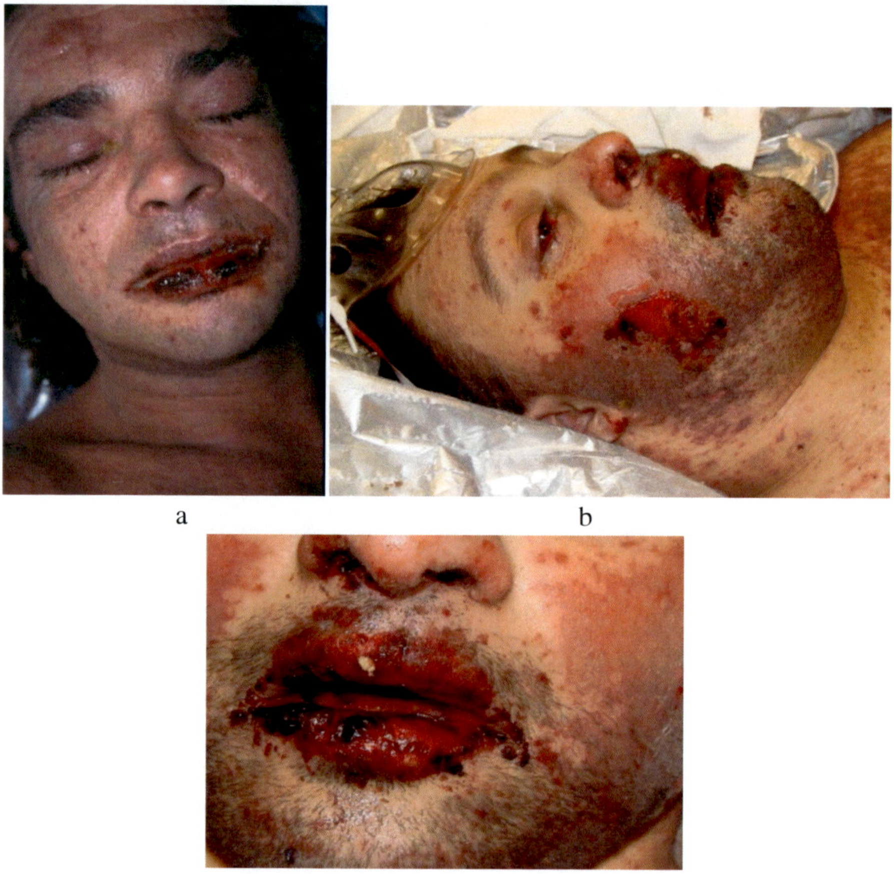

a b

c

Figure 2. Lip involvement in TEN. a - early erosive lesions. b, c- severe mucosal and epidermal involvement.

One case report of antibiotic-induced TEN corresponded to a patient who initially suffered from prolonged severe methotrexate (MTX)-induced pancytopenia without any detectable residual leukocytes including T lymphocytes and macrophages in the blood and skin [35]. This observation suggested that TEN keratinocytes were mainly responsible for their self-destruction without any evidence for the involvement of inflammatory cells.

Various pro-apoptotic systems are overexpressed by keratinocytes from the onset of TEN and in almost absence of inflammatory cells [17, 36]. In particular, tumor necrosis factor (TNF), and Fas receptor/Fas ligand (FasR/FasL, CD95R/CD95L) play apparently prominent roles [36]. In vitro studies demonstrated that TEN keratinocytes expressed lytically active FasL [19]. In addition, these cells express various pro-inflammatory cytokines and their corresponding receptors, as well as chemokines and their specific receptors, adhesion molecules and HLA-DR molecules. However, all these compounds are not typically overexpressed in TEN compared to healthy skin and various inflammatory dermatoses.

The calprotectin (L1-protein) complex is frequently expressed in the cytosol of both apparently uninvolved and clinically altered TEN epidermis [6, 37]. Calprotectin overexpression involves a calcium (Ca^{2+})-related process. Its presence in the apparently intact epidermis of TEN patients suggests that the increased Ca^{2+} concentration inside keratinocytes represents an incipient biologic event in TEN following the drug metabolite bioactivation.

The TEN pathomechanism is possibly regulated by other early events disturbing the cell cycle of proliferation. The model is provided by antifolate cytotoxic skin reactions (ACSR) induced by MTX closely mimicking the SJS/TEN presentation [38, 39]. It is framed as a hypothesis that the toxic drug metabolites in TEN block the cell cycle of proliferation in tissues where the metabolites are formed.

Secondary, nonspecific multisystemic involvements are frequent in TEN. Keratinocytes and inflammatory cells involved in the primary specific TEN processes produce large amounts of various pro-inflammatory cytokines that are released in the organism and contribute to general secondary symptoms including fever, synthesis of acute phase reactants, hematologic disturbances, and various effects on the internal organs.

Chapter 3

Immunological Mechanisms

TEN is considered to be an immune-mediated process by many authors. Indeed, rechallenging a former TEN patient with the same offending drug results in rapid recurrence of TEN [29]. By some aspects, TEN appears as an HLA class I-restricted, specific drug sensitivity, resulting in clonal expansion of CD8+ cytotoxic T lymphocytes (CTL). Cytotoxicity is mediated by CTL granzyme and death receptor (DR) and its ligand (DRL), likely FasL. Particular to TEN, amplification sequences involve further DRL expressions. FasL is likely to be particularly important, and TNF contributes via the TNF receptor 1 (TNF-R1) death pathway. Alternatively, a possible upregulation supervenes through the antiapoptotic TNF-R1-nuclear factor (NF) kB pathway. This process should proscribe treatments downregulating this pathway [41].

The links between drug-related immune reactions to the massive epidermal apoptosis, and the apoptotic pathways involved in TEN remain in part puzzling quandaries. Both lymphocytes and macrophages were extensively explored as potential direct or indirect cell mediators in the TEN pathogenesis [42]. Contrasting with most other dermatoses, inflammatory cells are particularly scanty in early TEN lesions. Several immunohistochemical studies were performed, and some discrepancies are still unresolved [43]. They are in part due to different timings of the tissue samplings. In general, $CD4^+$ T lymphocytes predominate in the upper dermis, whereas the relative composition of $CD8^+$ CTL and macrophages commonly prevails in the epidermis. Such immunological pattern appears particularly pertinent to drug-induced TEN.

A suggested pathological mechanism considers that TNF is in part responsible for cell death in TEN [33]. TNF is abundant in the TEN epidermis [41], as well as in mononuclear cells of blister fluid [44], peripheral blood mononuclear cells [45] and macrophages [46]. Soluble TNF (sTNF) and its receptor (sTNF-R) are present in blister fluid [47, 48]. Of note, the sTNF-R are more abundant in skin than in serum, suggesting an epidermal processing of TNF [48]. A possible source of TNF is necrotic keratinocytes releasing TNF or inducing its release from inflammatory cells. Anyway, TEN keratinocytes become apoptotic, and thus they are not expected to be at the origin of intrinsic high level activation of inflammatory cytokines.

It is notable that low levels of interleukin (IL)-1a, another primary inflammatory cytokine, are reported in TEN blister fluid compared to burns [49]. Whether any TNF release from keratinocytes is an active or passive process, TNF likely plays a pathogenic role in TEN.

Part II: Clinico-Pathologic Features

Chapter 4

Cutaneous and Mucosal Clinical Presentations

TEN is characterized by the extensive necrosis and detachment of large portions of the epidermis and mucosal epithelia. Both SJS and TEN present some similarities in their clinical presentation that, however, remain distinct in their extension.

TEN usually begins with nonspecific symptoms, including fever, cough, sore throat, malaise and burning eyes, followed after 1 to 3 days by skin and mucous membrane lesions. A burning painful erythematous rash starts symmetrically. It commonly prevails on the face, the upper part of the trunk and the proximal portions of the limbs. Most frequently, the initial skin lesions form a poorly defined macular exanthem with occasional purple purpuric centers (Figure 3). The lesions progressively extend and merge on the chest and back. They evolve to form raised confluent and flaccid blisters before epidermal sloughing. Such a sheet-like loss of epidermis typically occurs from the areas of confluent erythema. The flaccid blisters spread upon pressure, and Nikolsky sign is positive over large areas. Less frequently, the initial manifestation corresponds to an extensive scarlatiniform erythema. The ultimate extension of the lesions almost covering the whole TBSA is usually reached after 2 to 5 days, but sometimes in only a few hours. Occasionally, extension lasts longer, over a week or more.

The pale greyish necrotic epidermis is crumpled and wrinkled. Detachment of the full-thickness epidermis usually supervenes over pressure areas of the shoulders and buttocks, and on any traumatized site. Such a process leaves an uncovered purple-red oozing dermis.

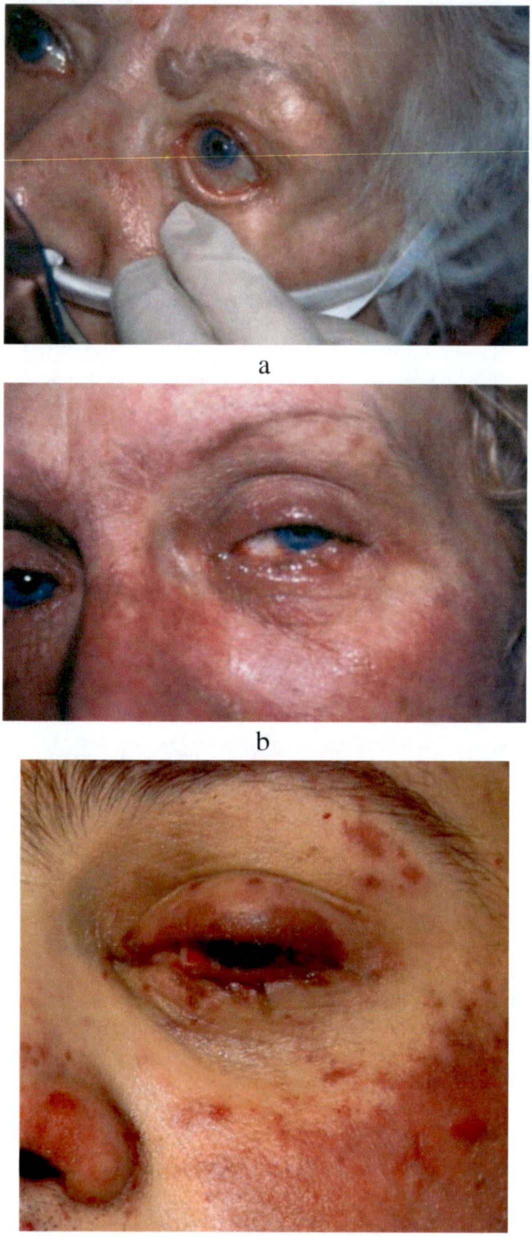

a

b

c

Figure 3. Ocular involvement in TEN. a - discrete conjunctival and lid involvement. b, c- severe lid involvement.

Almost, the entire skin surface and the eyes (Figure 3) are involved, with near to a generalized epidermal sloughing off. Of note, the hairy portion of the scalp is never involved. The extent of detachment of the epidermis should be appreciated daily, and expressed as the percentage of the TBSA involved. Wound pain is possibly assessed using a visual-analog scale (VAS) where 0 indicates absence of pain and 10 notifies the strongest and unbearable pain. The packing density of dermal dendrocytes is commonly increased (Figure 4).

Oral mucous membrane involvement is present in nearly all patients (85-95%). It frequently precedes the skin involvement, sometimes by 1 or 2 days. Early erosive lesions are frequently followed by widespread painful erosions. They cause crusted lips, increased salivation and impaired alimentation (Figure 2). In rare instances, severe mucosal alterations induce the formation of cysts in the secretory ducts of glands such as parotid [50]. Persistent mucosal ulcerations represent a rare complication of TEN [51, 52].

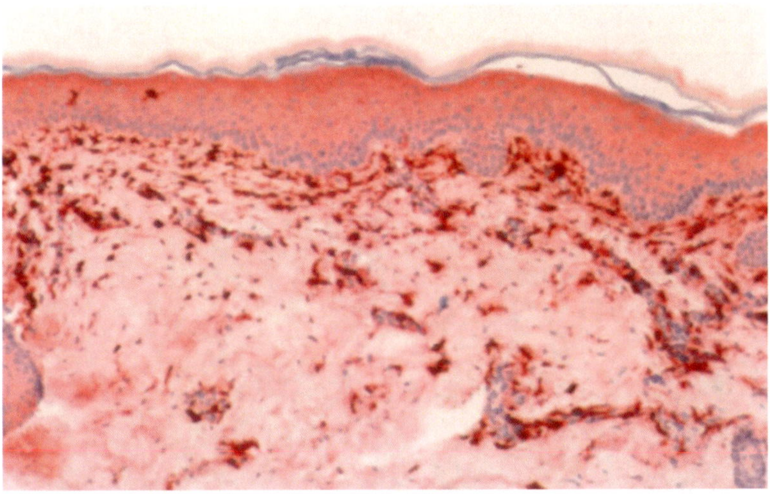

Figure 4. Factor XIIIa+ dermal dendrocytes in TEN.

Chapter 5

Extracutaneous Involvement

A prodromal phase combining fever, cough, sore throat, malaise and burning eyes often precedes the acute macular exanthem of TEN. In addition to the skin and oral mucosa alterations, TEN appears to specifically involve organs covered by a multistratified epithelium including the eyes (conjunctiva and cornea), esophagus, bronchial tree and vagina. Some segments of the excretory ducts of large salivary glands, and some foci of epidermoid metaplasia of the trachea and bronchioles exhibit a squamous multistratified epithelium, and they are prone to develop TEN erosions. Although, systemic involvement in TEN is acknowledged, it remains variable in its expression in organs.

5.1. Eye Involvement

The early and almost constant involvement of the eyes is noteworthy both in SJS and TEN [53-56]. Acute ocular involvement and chronic ocular sequelae are distinguished [57]. In some patients, the ocular presentation remains limited to conjunctivitis, but corneal erosions and other alterations are commonly present (Figure 3). In practice, a patient suffering from an widespread cutaneous rash and presenting with ocular involvement is possibly a SJS or TEN victim [53-59]. It is noteworthy that in absence of any ocular involvement, a skin rash is probably unrelated to TEN.

The acute ocular manifestations of SJS and TEN are characterized by inflammation of the entire ocular surface including the cornea, the bulbar/tarsal conjunctiva and the eyelid margin [55].

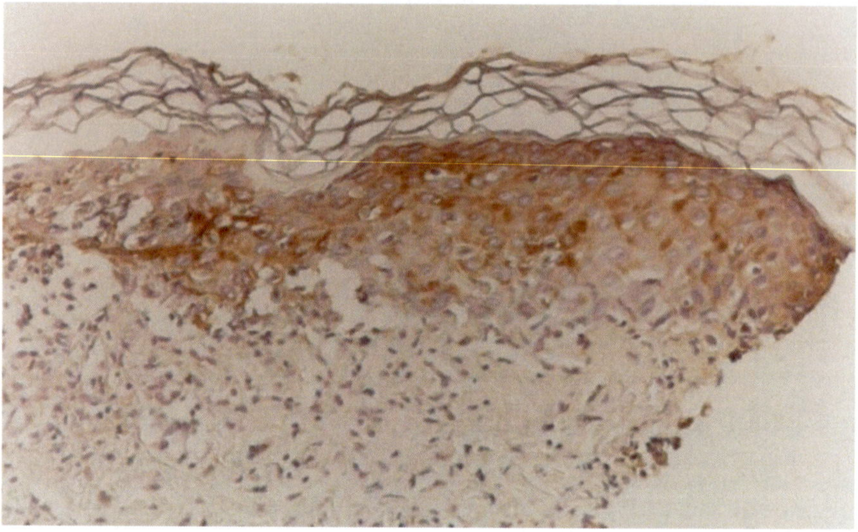

Figure 5. Epidermal necrolysis and detachement in TEN.

Ocular manifestations are roughly categorized as mild, moderate or severe. This classification allows a correlation between the initial ocular presentations and the outcome prognosis of the acute stage, but not the prediction of the evolution of the chronic sequel stage. Patients with TEN or in the SJS/TEN overlap group suffer from more frequent, but no more severe ocular involvement than patients with SJS. The severity of eye alterations in acute SJS and TEN does not closely match with the severity of skin involvement [60] (Figure 5) or systemic illness nor to the origin of the disease [60]. Most of the parameters influencing the global severity of TEN do not match with the severity of the acute phase of the eye involvement [54, 61].

Mild acute ocular involvement encompasses eyelid edema and skin denudation and desquamation. In addition, punctate epithelial erosions are present over less than 25% of the cornea, and/or mild conjunctival injection with redness, mucous discharge, and chemosis [61]. Conjunctival membranes and pseudomembranes are absent [61-63]. Such patients experience minor ocular discomfort with full resolution of ocular damages before hospital discharge.

Moderate acute ocular involvement includes epithelial defects up to 50% of the cornea, moderate conjunctival vascular dilations, and/or presence of conjunctival membranes or pseudomembranes. These patients keep almost normal vision, and nearly complete resolution of all active ocular changes is gained on discharge from the hospital.

Severe acute eye involvement combines epithelial defects and erosions over 50% of the cornea, severe conjunctival inflammation, and/or extensive conjunctival pseudomembranes or membranes [56]. The raw surfaces possibly lead to adhesion between the palpebral and bulbar conjonctiva corresponding to a symblepharon. Patients commonly complain from severe pain and photophobia. They suffer from extensive ocular inflammation with impaired vision. They require specific ongoing eye care after discharge. Eye involvement can be severe early in the disease, even before extensive skin sloughing has developed. Urgent ophthalmic advice should be part of the initial care of all SJS and TEN patients.

Because eye inflammation can progress quickly in the early time of illness, daily evaluations are recommended until there is evidence that no worsening is occurring. Detailed bedside examination should include the lid skin, the mucocutaneous junction and the tarsal conjunctiva. The entire ocular surface must be scrutinized using fluorescein staining and a handheld blue light ophthalmoscope in order to detect any epithelial defect or ulcer [62]. The severity of the acute ocular disease is the only acknowledged risk factor for late ocular complications in TEN patients [64].

The chronic ocular complications of SJS and TEN are mainly caused by prolonged ulcerations and relentless inflammation in the acute phase leading to scarring of the ocular surface. Ocular sequels represent the first long-term complications in patients with SJS and TEN. They cause major visual morbidity. They occur in up to one third of these patients who will suffer from a substantial lower overall health-related quality of life than the normal population. It is considered that about 87% of the patients with late ocular complications find it difficult to read, to drive at night, and to use a computer even for limited periods [62].

Scarring in the fornix obstructs the excretory ductules of the lacrimal glands. This problem leads to aqueous tear deficiency, and is one of the cause of the “dry eye syndrome”, representing the most common complication affecting up to 45-60% of the patients. However, other multifactorial causes result in dry eye in TEN patients. Inflammation and conjunctival necrosis in the acute phase promote goblet cells destruction and a decrease in mucin secretion. The corneal epithelium damages hinder tear adhesion. Epithelial integrity and mucin secretion play a prominent role in maintaining tear film stability. In addition, lipid tear deficiency caused by obliteration of the Meibomian gland orifices also promotes tear evaporation [60]. Eyelid complications and conjunctival retraction add a mechanical factor increasing tear evaporation. Dry eye is sufficient to cause lifelong, annoying irritation and to threaten vision [62].

During the healing process, scarring of the bulbar and forniceal conjunctivae potentially leads to adhesion called symblepharon or ankyloblepharon. Such a process occasionally obliterates the tear meniscus, interferes with aqueous tear flow, causes inadequate blinking/closure, and affects the ocular motility [62].

Scarring of the lid margins and tarsus occasionally leads to ectropion, entropion, trichiasis, distichiasis, Meibomian gland orifice metaplasia, punctual scarring and keratinization of the mucosal surface. These pathological changes can cause sight-threatening corneal complications by the ongoing trauma caused by friction from the lid malposition, the misdirected eyelashes and the scarred mucosal surfaces of the eyelids [62]. A strong correlation exists between the severity of lid margin keratinization, tarsal scarring and corneal involvement [60]. Some patients without any initial corneal lesion possibly develop corneal complications caused by the lid margin and tarsal conjunctival scarring.

Chronic ocular complications after SJS and TEN are not always direct consequences of palpebral conjunctival or corneal scarring. Late (a few month to years) surface failure possibly occurs as a consequence of recurrent conjunctival inflammation unrelated to mechanical irritation or to dryness.

Ocular lesions need special attention and daily examinations by an ophthalmologist because they carry a high risk of sequels. In the initial acute phase, redness and soreness of the eyes are conspicuous. Pseudomembranous conjunctival erosions are common and associated with a tendency to form synechiae between the eyelids and conjunctiva during the healing phase. Keratitis and corneal erosions are less frequent. A sicca syndrome possibly develops in a second step.

5.2. Respiratory Tract Involvement

A specific acute respiratory involvement occurs in about 25-30 % of TEN patients. Fibre optic bronchoscopy reveals sloughing of bronchial epithelium in proximal airways [65]. Clinical respiratory involvement is a worrisome event [66, 67]. Hyperventilation is common with mild to severe hypoxemia. Such a condition should be suspected when dyspnea, bronchial hypersecretion, marked hypoxemia and expectorations of bronchial mucosal casts develop during the early TEN stage. The parenchymal lung remains commonly uninvolved, but the necrolytic process occasionally reaches the tracheobronchial epithelium with a possible fatal outcome.

In survivors, slightly protracted pulmonary complications, generally between day 7 and 15, include pulmonary edema, atelectasia, bacterial pneumonia and adult respiratory distress syndrome (ARDS) [65]. Such protracted complications result from metabolic disturbances without prominent epithelial detachment. Hypersecretion is characterized by fluid, yellowish, non-purulent spittle, suggesting plasma exudation across the altered bronchial epithelial barrier. Respiratory symptoms related to bronchial and tracheal detachment develop rapidly, generally within 4 days, after the onset of mucocutaneous detachment. Bronchial biopsies confirm the extensive epithelial necrosis of trachea and bronchi.

This process is accompanied by minute inflammation. Inflammatory cells infiltrating respiratory mucosae consist of lymphocytes and monocytes, in a pattern similar to that found in TEN cutaneous lesions, and suggesting similar pathomechanisms. Respiratory involvement in TEN is apparently not correlated with the extent of epidermal detachment or with some specific offending drugs. The basic mechanisms responsible for bronchial and tracheal necrolysis in TEN remain unknown. However, airway sloughing off and skin detachment appear almost synchronous, and they both regenerate over the same timing, what further suggest specific TEN bronchial and tracheal epithelial involvement.

Delayed unspecific pulmonary complications develop in most of survivors following bronchial epithelial detachment, but only in about 25% of TEN patients free of early pulmonary manifestations. These alterations occur generally in the second week after admission, and they mainly consist of pulmonary edema, atelectasia and bacterial pneumonitis. In patients devoid of early specific involvement, bronchoscopy reveals a normal appearing respiratory mucosae and histopathology confirms the absence of tracheal or bronchial epithelial necrosis.

Although alterations of the broncho-pulmonary epithelial barrier are suspected in patients with bronchial mucosal detachment, fluid overload appears involved more frequently in pulmonary edema since TEN treatment requires abundant fluid supplies.

5.3. Gastrointestinal Tract Involvement

Disseminated involvement of the gastrointestinal mucosa affects some TEN patients. The esophagus epithelium is commonly involved tissue. When present, disseminated erosions of the pharynx and esophagus lead to dysphagia and occasionally to bleeding [68,69]. Spontaneous evolution possibly results in esophageal strictures. The prevalence of esophageal involvement is grossly underestimated, because oropharyngeal dysphagia commonly masks esophageal dysphagia. Endoscopy shows diffuse erosions macroscopically indistinguishable from peptic esophagitis. A mucosal biopsy specimen from the esophagus discloses a pattern of intraepithelial inflammatory cells with necrosis of individual epithelial cells, similar to the changes in incipient skin lesions.

Overt intestinal symptoms are uncommon, but they present as severe lesions when present [70, 71]. They are reminiscent of ulcerative [72] or pseudomembranous colitis. A profuse protein-rich diarrhea increases fluid losses and hypoalbuminemia. Histopathologic features resemble those of the intestinal lesions of GVHD.

A few cases of liver damages and acute pancreatitis have been reported in association with TEN. An increase in serum amylase and lipase is present during the first few days, without any other evidence of pancreatic involvement [73]. The few computed tomographic scans in patients with raised serum amylase levels looked normal.

5.4. Kidney Involvement

Renal involvement is prevalent in TEN patients [74]. Proteinuria, renal tubular enzyme excretion, and microalbuminuria are frequent, indicating both proximal tubular involvement and secondary effects on glomerular structure [75]. Functional tubular dysfunction possibly results from nonspecific factors including stress, hypovolemia and low cardiac output. Because various cytokines exert direct toxic effects on several kidney structures, the tubular damage and the increased glomerular activity are possibly related to the nephrotoxic effects of cytokines involved in TEN.

There is about a 20% frequency of acute renal failure with a need for dialysis (3%), and a risk for hypokalemia (7%) in SJS and TEN patients. Sepsis, associated drugs such as allopurinol, nonsteroidal anti-inflammatory drugs (NSAIDS) and antibiotics, chronic kidney disease and hypoalbuminuria are independent risk factors for acute renal failure in SJS and TEN patients.

5.5. Pregnancy

SJS and TEN have an impact in gynecology [16, 76, 77]. In rare instances, TEN develops simultaneously in a mother and her fetus [78-80]. The placenta in TEN women only shows mild chorioamnionitis [80]. By contrast, the disease is generally lethal for the fetus. Three mechanisms of mother-to-fetus TEN transmission are possible, namely: (a) common defects in detoxification pathways of reactive drug metabolites, (b) similar genetic predispositions to TEN development, and (c) presence of drug-specific cytotoxic T lymphocytes (CTL) first present in the mother's blood, and next circulating in the fetus bloodstream.

5.6. Sepsis

The risk of infectious complications is common in TEN patients, particularly those due to Gram-positive micro-organisms including *Staphylococcus aureus*, and later during the hospital course, to Gram-negative bacteria such as *Pseudomonas aeruginosa*. Since over half of TEN-related deaths result from sepsis, control of the skin bacterial and fungal colonization and infection are critical aspects of TEN management.

Fever is usual even in absence of infection in TEN patients, and it occasionally persists until complete skin healing. Of note, a sudden hypothermia is more indicative of severe sepsis than fever. Asthenia, skin pain, anxiety, agitation and confusion are commonly prominent. They often herald hemodynamic complications of sepsis. Over half of TEN-related deaths result from sepsis. Bacteria (*Staphylococcus* spp.) and fungi (*Candida albicans*, *Mucor* spp.) are the most frequent aggressors [10-12].

5.6.1. Staphylococcal Infection

Among a variety of Gram-positive microorganisms, the different *Staphylococcus* spp. are classified according to specific combinations of phenotypic characteristics and DNA relatedness. The clinically most important bacteria is *S. aureus*. The chief sites of *S. aureus* colonization are the anterior nostrils, perineum, axillae, and toe webs. Typical staphylococcal infections consist of pustules, impetiginous lesions and folliculitis, as well as furuncles and carbuncles. A smear examination reveals the presence of Gram-positive cocci arranged as irregular large clusters. Later during the hospital course, Gram-negative bacteria such as *Pseudomonas aeruginosa* potentially interfere with the TEN outcome.

5.6.2. Candida Infection

Candida spp. are dimorphic yeasts of the normal human biocene. Various *Candida* spp. are present inside the mouth and digestive tract in about half of the population, and they colonize the vagina in up to 20% of asymptomatic women. They normally remain harmless colonizers of the mucosae. Dimorphism between bastoconidia yeasts and filamentous pseudohyphae is characteristic of this organism. Blastoconidia forms are the dominant aspect of hematogenous dissemination, whereas mycelial growth of elongated hyphae is considered the dominant presentation of tissue invasive infections.

Candida spp. adherence and colonization of oropharyngeal and gastrointestinal mucosae are under the influence of several conditions favoring these organisms over other agents of the regular resident microbial flora. Systemic infection often originates from these sites, as well as from the vaginal mucosa and skin.

Disseminated candidiasis refers to the migration of yeasts to other sites where they are not regular commensal organisms. Most systemic Candida infections develop from transient fungemia in an hematogenous dissemination to one or more organs. The hematogeneous spread of *Candida* spp. leads to various organ involvements, including pulmonary infections, meningitis, encephalitis, endophthalmitis, hepatitis, peritonitis, endocarditis. Almost all yeast-infected patients are febrile.

In TEN patients, the bypass of epithelial barriers and the presence of indwelling intravenous catheters carry a predilection for *Candida* fungemia. Hyperglycemia resulting from hyperalimentation, and presence of oral mucositis and esophagitis are particularly prone of the dissemination process.

Demonstration of the yeast in lesional tissue or at sites not commonly colonized by *Candida* spp. supports the diagnosis of candidiasis. Cytologic examination of fluids or epithelial scrapings, and tissue biopsies of affected organs represent valuable diagnostic procedures. Colonization and superficial infections of the oropharynx, vagina, and skin are rapidly confirmed by scraping the surface epithelial cells from lesions for demonstrating the characteristic hyphae, pseudohyphae, and blastoconidia yeasts of *Candida* spp. *Candida* spp. are best visualized with special stains, either periodic acid-Schiff (PAS) or Gomori methenamine silver (GMS).

The characteristic histopathology of candidiasis is an acute inflammatory infiltrate of polynuclear leukocytes forming micro-abscesses about a mass of blastoconidia, pseudohyphae, and necrotic debris. Pseudohyphae invade the proximal boundary tissue.

In systemic Candida infections of visceral organs, small abscesses are typically composed of both neutrophils and mononuclear cells. Because hematogenous dissemination is the usual route of infection, a vascular distribution or vasculitic pattern is commonly present.

Although multiple visceral organs are typically affected in disseminated candidiasis, the skin is involved in 10-15% of patients. The lesions exhibit varied sizes (2 to 20 mm) and numbers, but only a few are usually present. Occasionally, they are generalized or, more typically located on the extremities. Most often, they correspond to erythematous, maculo-papular to nodular lesions with a pale center. Several other presentations are possible including purpuric or pustular lesions.

Ocular candidiasis manifestations are responsible for downgrading of visual acuity, blurred vision, pain, photophobia, and scotomas. Endophthalmitis is accompanied by white fluffy exudates of chorioretinitis, vitreous hemorrhages, iritis, and conjunctivitis. The presence of ocular lesions is commonly associated with multi-organ involvement, and up to 50% of candidemia patients manifest obvious ocular lesions.

5.6.3. Mucor Infection

Mucor spp. are ubiquitous molds that occasionally behave as opportunistic pathogens. TEN represents a condition at risk for developing a mucormycosis [11]. Invasive mucormycosis occurs when macrophages are ineffective in the control of the disease. Most often, the infection begins in the nose and paranasal sinuses before disseminating to the head and elsewhere.

5.7. Multisystemic and Late Internal Complications

A secondary multisystemic involvement is quite frequent in TEN. Rhabdomyolysis [81], and hematologic disturbances (leukopenia, anemia, neutropenia disseminated intravascular coagulation) are possible [82]. Most of the metabolic failures of internal organs probably result from the primary destruction of large areas of stratified epithelia leading to seemingly cytokine storms.

Long-term internal complications are rare in TEN survivors. They encompass intestinal ulcers, diffuse heterotopic calcifications [83], chronic renal failure, and pulmonary complications (persistent reduction in carbon monoxide diffusing capacity, obstructive bronchitis/bronchiolitis, bronchiectasis) [84]. The most common long-term morbidities in TEN survivors involve the skin (80-100%), the eyes (25 to 55%), the nails (35%), and the oral/vulvovaginal mucosae (10-15%) [85-90]. Numerous post-TEN complications, especially chronic eye involvement and dental alterations [91], significantly impair the overall quality of life, emphasizing the need for long-term follow-up

Chapter 6

Histopathology

6.1. Skin

It is mandatory to examine a skin biopsy from each case of SCAR. The biopsy has a medicolegal value and is important in the event of a lawsuit. In such a context, the diagnosis of TEN usually seems to be clinically evident. Yet, nearly half of the referred patients for a TEN suspicion suffer from another disease. The differential diagnosis is sometimes difficult, and an early biopsy is the only confirmatory diagnostic test [92].

The initial TEN lesions are characterized by the presence of vacuolar changes at the dermo-epidermal junction, associated with a sparse cell infiltrate admixed to scattered or clustered dyskeratotic (apoptotic) keratinocytes. Histopathologically, TEN presents with apoptotic/necrotic keratinocytes in either a widespread distribution or full-thickness necrosis of the epidermis. Vacuolization leading to subepidermal blistering is present in the basal membrane zone. A sparse superficial, often perivascular lymphohistiocytic infiltrate is present in the upper dermis [93].

It is framed as an hypothesis that the causative drug possibly generates specific toxic metabolite(s) by epithelial cells. This process in turn likely exerts cytotoxic effects on keratinocytes in the neighborhood. This event is possibly mediated by the combination of (a) an increased accumulation of intracellular Ca^{2+}, (b) the induction of reactive oxygen species (ROS) including nitric oxide (NO), and (c) the activation of both CD95 and TNF [36, 94]. Another possible pathomechanism is ascribed to lymphocytes, particularly CD8+ CTL and natural killer (NK) cells infiltrating the epidermis and acting through the perforin/granzyme B pathway, and more importantly by granulysin peptide [95]. In addition, macrophages and Factor XIIIa+ dermal dendrocytes (DD) appear to exert some pathogenic role in TEN [96, 97]. Complex interactions linking such cytotoxic effects likely participate in the massive apoptosis/necrosis of keratinocytes.

Apoptosis/necrosis of keratinocytes is a prominent finding in SJS and TEN. Other epidermal features include focal liquefaction/degeneration of basal cells, spongiosis, and exocytosis of scanty set of mononuclear cells. With evolving lesions, distinct histopathologic zones corresponding to the observed clinical changes are disclosed. Thus, the histopathologic changes present in the lesion reflect a dynamic evolving process. Early erythematous papules and the enlarging border of evolving macular lesions share similar histopathologic signs. They include apoptosis of individual epidermal cells, prominent papillary dermal edema, vascular dilations with endothelial cell swelling and apoptosis [98], as well as a scanty perivascular mononuclear cell infiltrate. Within the dusky center of macular lesions, where the epidermal injury is more severe, extensive epithelial necrosis, liquefaction degeneration of the basal cell layer, and swelling of the papillary dermis are prominent. The necrotic epidermis forms the roof of subepidermal blisters. The number of neutrophils and eosinophils in the inflammatory infiltrate is quite small, especially in early lesions. There is no evidence for sign of vasculitis.

The dermatopathologic changes observed in SJS and TEN reflect the severe epidermal injury observed clinically. Necrosis of the basal cell layer with incontinence of melanin pigment and dermal colloid bodies are common features. Extensive epithelial necrosis and microscopic subepidermal blister formation are found in most specimens, and complete epidermal detachment occurs in severe lesions. Mononuclear cells are dispersed in the upper dermis and epidermis, although the infiltrate is commonly sparse. The timing of a biopsy during the evolution of the disease greatly influences the histopathology.

6.2. Eye

Pathological alterations of the corneal epithelium in the early acute stage of TEN demonstrate vacuolisation of the basal keratinocyte cytoplasm, and occasional apoptotic keratinocytes without evidence of intraepithelial CTL infiltration or necrosis at this stage [60, 99]. This corresponds to similar changes observed in the skin, and means that a cytokine-mediated mechanism response contributes to the initial insult. This process precedes CTL infiltration which is then associated with poor healing and erosions. These cytokines are produced by the corneal epithelial cells themselves or are derived from conjunctival tissue. The key cytokines involved in surface repair and damage include TNF, IL-1 and matrix metalloproteinases (MMP). Limbal stem cell deficiency possibly occurs with corneal lesions [100]. Neutrophils are also involved [101].

During chronic ocular sequels, clusters of CD8+ CTL infiltrate the corneal epithelium. The cytopathic effect of the intraepithelial CTL manifests as discohesion, vacuolar changes and condensation of the epithelial eosinophilic cytoplasm suggesting apoptotic changes.

Chapter 7

Proteomic Kinetic Analysis

Proteomic analyses provide a unique opportunity to explore disease-related changes present in the protein content of selected body fluids. A unique exploratory study was performed in TEN [102]. The findings correlated with dermatopathologic evidence, indicated that GSH transferase p is involved in the oxidative stress present in TEN epidermis. The monocyte differentiation antigen CD14 and myeloperoxidase documented the macrophage activation. The pro-inflammatory S100-A8 protein seemingly originates from activated keratinocytes and/or macrophages. The global proteomic findings are in line with immunohistochemical findings, and they support the prominent involvement of keratinocytes and macrophages in the TEN pathomechanism.

Chapter 8

Differential Diagnosis

A series of diseases should be considered in the differential diagnosis of SCAR [103, 104]. These conditions are rare, but some of them possibly cause severe morbidity and have a demise issue.

In the SJS or TEN bullous stage, the main clinical differential diagnoses include the staphylococcal scalded skin syndrome (SSSS), the acute generalized exanthematous pustulosis (AGEP) and the generalized bullous fixed drug eruption [94]. The Drug Rash with Eosinophilia and Systemic Symptoms (DRESS) syndrome has to be considered although blistering is not the rule in this entity.

8.1. Erythema Multiforme

Erythema multiforme (EM) corresponds to an acute self-limited skin disease. Its onset is abrupt. The lesions are symmetrically distributed on the extremities and they exhibit typical concentric target-like lesions. Early EM presents as red maculo-papules evolving over several days to form annular lesions corresponding to an erythematous raised and palpable rim surrounding a dusky center. Typical target-like lesions exhibit at least three different areas characterized by two concentric rings encircling a central disc. More unusual lesions show only two zones. Each lesion persists at each given site for days, but typically the morphology varies over time. Because of the absence of specific diagnostic clues, EM is diagnosed largely based on its clinical features. Consequently, there is a possible wide range of disorders diagnosed as EM. Such a rather confusing heterogeneity is present in the medical literature regarding EM.

A distinction was formerly offered between the mild afebrile EM minor from the more severe EM major, usually febrile, with involvement of several mucous membranes. This latter condition corresponds nowadays to SJS.

EM lesions predominantly develop in young males, without any ethnic predilection [105]. Lesions are often confined to mucosae and cutaneous acral sites. EM often corresponds to a distant reaction accompanied by some infectious diseases, most notably those due to some HSV types. Recurrent EM probably accounts for a number of cases. They do not necessarily follow every episode of recurrent HSV, and clinical evidence of HSV infection does not always antedate every EM episode. Bullous EM has been reported as a rare complication of *Mycoplasma pneumoniae* infection [106]. No association is recognized with HIV infection [105], and a drug reaction is rarely involved in EM [107]. EM skin lesions occasionally occur with increased density at sites of recent sun exposure. Photo-accentuation of skin lesions is characterized by the combination of an almost confluent erythema developed at sites of a recent mild sunburn, and a sharply demarcated decrease in the density of skin lesions on light-protected skin.

The duration of each EM episode ranges from 1 to 4 weeks, with a median duration lasting about 3 weeks. The onset of skin lesions is abrupt, and the majority of skin and mucosal lesions appear within the first 72 hours of the illness. During the eruptive phase, the patient experiences itching, burning, or prickling sensations of the skin, but these symptoms gradually subside. A few patients experience new crops of papules every few days during the course of one episode of EM. More rarely, a prolonged overlapping series of lesional recurrences produces the pattern of continuous EM. Most patients with EM are febrile throughout the course of the disease, do not experience other systemic symptoms, and recover completely. Many episodes of EM are so mild that symptomatic care is all that is required.

In EM, the oral mucosa is the only mucosal site likely involved. Oral lesions typically correspond to erosions on the gingivae, labial mucosa, buccal mucosa and tongue. They occur in about 25% of cases. Usually fewer than a dozen of discrete erosions are present, but in some patients erosions extend over most of the gingival surfaces. Oral lesions are commonly accompanied by tender cervical lymphadenopathies. Mucosal lesions usually appear simultaneously to the skin lesions, but occasionally precede or follow the onset of skin lesions by several days.

The mononuclear cell infiltrate is commonly denser in EM than in TEN [46]. Human leukocyte antigen (HLA) typing indicates that an increased likelihood of developing EM is associated with the presence of certain HLA types related to ethnicity.

A series of diagnostic criteria bring greater selectivity and confidence in the diagnosis of EM: (a) the illness must be acute and self-limited or episodic, (b) the duration of a single episode must be less than 6 weeks, (c) skin lesions must be discrete, fixed, lasting for more than 7 days, generally round in shape, and symmetrically distributed, (d) at least some of the lesions must evolve to form concentric zones of color compatible with target lesions, and (e) the histopathological presentation should be indicative [46] without evidence of leucocytoclastic vasculitis or neutrophil predominance in the inflammatory infiltrate. Cases fulfilling these criteria, with mucous membrane involvement remaining discrete or limited to the mouth, likely correspond to EM, while those with widespread cutaneous lesions and involvement of two or more mucosal surfaces are classified as SJS.

8.2. Stevens-Johnson Syndrome

SJS, the SJS/TEN intermediate condition and TEN are considered as a spectrum of diseases differing only by the extent in epidermal alterations. They exhibit flat target-like patches and/or macules. Whereas EM lesions tend to be raised and target-like, lesions of the SJS and TEN spectrum appear flat and widespread [5]. SJS was initially termed "a new eruptive fever with stomatitis and ophthalmia". For years, SJS was considered as part of the EM spectrum, corresponding to EM major. This concept is now outdated. Only a close correlation between clinical, etiologic and histopathologic features allows to properly distinguish EM, SJS and TEN [46].

Circumscribed SJS lesions, as well as early TEN macules are small and of irregular shape, deeply erythematous or purpuric with a necrotic or blistering centre. Some initial SJS and TEN lesions are covered by blisters [5]. SJS is defined by the extent of blistering not exceeding over 10% of the TBSA. The skin surrounding the blisters is commonly erythematous and tender, and some blisters become hemorrhagic. Blister roofs are commonly shed, uncovering erythematous and tender erosions. When epidermal shedding occurs over large areas of skin, the clinical aspect overlaps with that of TEN. SJS lesions often evolve rapidly into large erythematous areas with blister formation and epidermal necrosis.

At least two mucosal surfaces are involved in SJS, with the mouth being affected in nearly all cases. Most SJS patients have lesions of the mouth and eyes. Other involved mucosal areas are the genital mucous membranes. In approximately 40% of SJS patients, all three mucosal sites are involved. Swelling, redness, burning, tingling, and tenderness of the lips and oral mucosa often represent the first signs of mucosal involvement. They precede or follow the onset of skin lesions. In many instances, erythematous areas and transient blisters on the mucosa quickly evolve into large erosions with swelling and crusting.

The SJS patients typically develop hemorrhagic crusts over the lips, along with a malodorous pseudomembrane of necrotic epithelium and a purulent exudates. Severe oral pain, with disabilities in eating, swallowing, and talking, commonly develop with hypersalivation and trismus. The ocular involvement in SJS includes redness, swelling, erosions, and a purulent discharge, accompanied by severe pain and photophobia. Pseudomembrane over conjunctival surfaces is commonly formed. Genital involvement is characterized by pain and erythema, followed by blisters and erosions. In women this involvement presents as a severely painful vulvovaginitis, while in men, painful erosions of the urethral meatus accompanied by a purulent discharge frequently develop. Urethral or vaginal bleeding occasionally develops when the mucosa is denuded. Anal erosions are infrequent, and other mucosal sites such as the esophagus, nasopharynx, trachea, or bronchi remain usually unaffected.

The course of SJS is prolonged, lasting for up to 6 weeks. The duration of the disease is directly related to the extent of the cutaneous surface and to the number of mucosal sites involved. Although patients with SJS experience the same cutaneous signs as those with EM, systemic symptoms including fever, malaise, arthralgias and myalgias, are commonly prominent and persistent in SJS.

No cause other than drugs is commonly recognized at the origin of SJS and TEN. Of the drugs involved in SJS, antibiotics, sulfonamides, nonsteroidal anti-inflammatory agents, and anticonvulsants stand out. Accordingly, any diagnosis of post-infectious SJS should probably be revisited as a major expression of EM. The clinical distinction between SJS and TEN is roughly established by the extent of epidermal sloughing. In SJS, less than 30% of TBSA is affected, accompanied by a moderate involvement of the mucosae.

By contrast TEN eroded lesions extend over 10% of TBSA with an extensive destruction of mucosal epithelia.

In addition to clinical and etiologic differences [106], the EM, SJS and TEN conditions are clearly distinguished by histopathology. EM presents as an inflammatory T cell-rich dermatitis contrasting with the inflammatory cell-poor SJS and TEN lesions [46]. On regular dermatopathology, confluent necrotic keratinocytes are the hallmark of TEN. The dermo-epidermal junction exhibits changes ranging from vacuolar alterations to subepidermal blisters. The lymphoid cell infiltrate commonly remains superficial and rare [93]. T lymphocytes usually predominate during the early phase of the disease, while macrophages and Factor XIIIa+ dermal dendrocytes rapidly predominate during the next few days [36, 93]. In addition, a strong TNF immunoreactivity is typically found in TEN keratinocytes [36]. Some other molecular markers represent ancillary parameters distinguishing EM from SJS and TEN. For instance, serum IL-13 levels are increased in patients with SJS and TEN, but not in those with EM [107].

SJS is a serious systemic illness with major complications. Fluid loss and leakage of electrolytes and proteins from the denuded skin and mucosa mimic that observed in burn patients. Skin lesions are often colonized by pathogen bacteria, and occasionally they become secondarily infected. Most skin lesions resolve without scarring, but leave post-inflammatory hyperpigmentation. By contrast, some other severely denuded areas of skin heal with hypopigmentation, scar formation, and contractures similar to the features seen after deep burns.

SJS complications are determined largely by the extent and severity of the damages to the skin and mucosal surfaces. Limitations to eat and drink because of oro-pharyngeal pain promote dehydration, and contribute to prolonged debilitation. Morbidity is prominent when a pseudomembrane develops on mucosal surfaces and leads to scarring. Such a process is especially damaging in the eye, leading to dryness sensations, immobile eyelids, symblepharon, entropion, trichiasis, corneal scarring, and permanent visual impairment. Lacrimal scarring, anterior uveitis, and panophthalmia are other rare ocular complications. Mouth and lip lesions usually heal without sequels, but scarring at other mucosal sites leads to esophageal strictures, anal strictures, vaginal stenosis, and urethral meatal stenosis. Damage to the respiratory tract resulting in persistent cough and pleural effusions possibly develop. Urinary retention, hematuria, and anuria result from dehydration and genitourinary injury. Myocarditis, pneumothorax, gastrointestinal bleeding, hepatitis and nephritis are unusual SJS complications. Rarely, the patient becomes progressively obtunded and develop coma and seizures.

Mortality rates (1-3 %) remain limited in SJS [4]. However, when associated with pneumonia, the mortality rate is increased. Likewise, mortality in cases with characteristics of SJS/TEN approaches 10-50%.

8.3. Graft-Versus-Host Reaction

Grade IV acute graft-versus-host reaction (GVHR) commonly resembles TEN [108]. Despite clinical, histopathologic and immunohistochemical criteria, an undisputable distinction between some cases of TEN and lymphocyte-depleted GVHR remains difficult to establish [109-111]. In fact, a close look at a clinicopathological correlation is required [111]. Attention must be paid to the biopsy timing, and to any possible eye alterations. For instance, the ocular involvement is typically found in most of the TEN patients, but in only 10% of those with severe GVHR. The onset of the TEN clinical signs is generally more dramatic than in GVHR, particularly in the immunosuppressed patients with GVHR. The presence of some extracutaneous involvements (liver, gut) often helps supporting the diagnosis of GVHR.

The density of the inflammatory infiltrate in the skin is generally as low in drug-induced TEN as in treated GVHR. Immunohistochemistry helps reaching the diagnosis by increasing the detection sensitivity of the epithelial alterations and the nature of the inflammatory cell infiltrate [111]. It must be stressed that a restricted follicular involvement is common in GVHR, but is often absent in TEN. At the difference with TEN, cytokeratin (CK)-15+ keratinocytes appear to be specifically targeted in GVHR [112, 113].

GVHR and the effect of imiquimod therapy show some resemblance in the aspect of epidermal lesions and the nature and density of the inflammatory cell infiltrate [114].

8.4. Cytotoxic Drug Reactions

Some cytostatic drugs, particularly MTX, are occasionally responsible for extensive epithelial necrosis. As a rule, the TEN causative drug itself is not a direct toxic compound for the organs, but rather an idiosyncratic alteration of the drug metabolism is evoked inside keratinocytes [6, 9]. The presumed toxic metabolites are thought to be responsible for apoptosis of keratinocytes. In addition, CD8+, CD56+ CTL and macrophages are involved in the pathomechanism of epithelial damages. These inflammatory cells possibly act as primary offenders to keratinocytes rather than acting as passive bystanders.

In specific instances, particularly following antifolate administration including MTX and pemetrexed (PTX) for cancer chemotherapy, focal or widespread epidermal necrosis occurs. The skin reaction is presumably due to a direct massive cytotoxic effect by the drug [38, 39, 115-118]. The various clinical aspects of such adverse events were tentatively coined antifolate cytotoxic skin reaction (ACSR) [39].

MTX is occasionally associated with severe ACSR including life-threatening conditions [38, 39, 115, 116, 119-122]. In addition, acral erythema represents a typical or suggestive finding [123, 124]. The most severe MTX-related ACSR look alike regular TEN or SJS. However, the pathobiology appears quite different. Clearly, the sublethal and lethal signs of MTX-related ACSR are present in both keratinocytes and endothelial cells. They seemingly result from a block in the S phase of cell proliferation. Notably, Factor XIIIa+ DD are plump and even show some ballooning [125].

PTX administration is commonly followed by certain adverse reactions [126-128]. These manifestations include myelosuppression characterized by anemia, neutropenia and thrombocytopenia. In addition, various digestive tract dysfunctions are commonly present, including nausea, vomiting, diarrhea, constipation, anorexia, stomatitis or oral erosions. In oncologic practice, the dose-limiting toxicity of PTX is determined by the myelosuppression although certain other non-hematologic toxicities occur before myelosuppression is reached. PTX-related ACSR are commonly referred to as “cutaneous rash” without any other identification or specificity. Among the identified ACSR, life-threatening conditions including TEN or TEN-like presentations have been reported [117, 129, 130]. Of note, the combination of cisplatin to PTX has been reported to suppress in part PTX toxicity. When both drugs are given on the same dosing day, the adverse effects are less than those encountered when both drugs are administered on separate conservative days.

8.5. Staphylococcal Scaled Skin Syndrome

SSSS is a specific exfoliative and bullous skin disease resulting from the effect of the exfoliative-toxin-producing *Staphylococcus aureus* [131]. Most often a purulent infection precedes in the upper respiratory tract, but any other staphylococcal infection can play a similar initiating role. The epidermolytic toxin-producing strains often belong to phage group 2. SSSS mainly affects infants and children. Skin lesions range from localized bullae resembling bullous impetigo to a diffuse exfoliative condition resulting from systemic toxemia. Bullae are typically thinner than in TEN, and the Nickolsky sign is present. Mucosal involvements and ocular lesions are not present in SSSS.

The initial lesions commonly appear on the face and the major body folds, spreading later to the trunk and the extremities. The erythematous macules are tender to the touch and exhibit a rough, sand paper-like texture. Within hours, spontaneous detachment of the skin takes place in large sheets. The blisters are fragile and transient, leaving large areas of exfoliative erythroderma. Bacterial toxemia, excessive water loss and electrolytic imbalance represent a risk for hemodynamic shock and fatal issue.

It is most important for the patient to rapidly establish the possible diagnosis of SSSS from a Tzanck smear and a histopathologic examination. Epidermal sloughing results from intraepidermal cleavage located inside the granular layer. Scattered necrotic keratinocytes are admixed to lymphocytes and neutrophils. Immunohistochemistry confirms that TEN differs from SSSS by both the absence of CD15+ granulocytes and a stronger expression of the pro-apoptotic CD95 antigen in the epidermis [131]. The cytologic examination of a Tzanck smear of denuded areas shows typical epithelial cells of the stratum granulosum. The initial staphylococcal infection is present at the distant focal site. Nose, throat, conjunctiva and any impetigo area should be swabbed for bacterial culture.

8.6. Acute Generalized Exanthematous Pustulosis

AGEP is an uncommon cutaneous eruption that is most often induced by drugs, acute *Enterovirus* infections, or mercury poisoning. It is characterized by acute extensive formation of nonfollicular sterile pustules dispersed on an erythematous background. This condition is associated with fever and neutropenia [132]. Involvement of T cells in drug-induced AGEP is possible [133, 134]. The histopathology and immunohistochemistry of acute AGEP are quite typical. They are characterized by a massive inflammatory cell infiltrate composed predominantly of neutrophils collected in spongiform subcorneal or intraepidermal pustules, and admixed to T cells, both in subepidermal and perivascular locations [133].

8.7. Generalized Fixed Drug Eruption

In multilocular or generalized fixed drug eruption (FDE), large irregularly distributed purplish-livid color patches appear faintly discernible even after confluence. Mucous membrane involvement and general symptoms are rare. Hence, the disease takes a milder course than SJS and TEN. Histopathology shows a more pronounced inflammatory cell reaction and a marked edema and swelling of the papillary dermis compared to SJS and TEN.

8.8. Drug Rash with Eosinophilia and Systemic Symptoms

DRESS syndrome, formerly called drug-induced hypersensitivity syndrome, is a potential fatal drug-induced disease. It combines a widespread erythematous eruption, fever, lymphadenopathies, hepatitis, as well as hematologic alterations including eosinophilia and atypical lymphocytes [135]. Blistering of the cutaneous lesions rarely occurs. The multivisceral involvement differentiates DRESS from TEN. In TEN contrasting with DRESS, eosinophilia is absent, and there is only slight kidney and liver involvements. Mucosal and ocular lesions are rare and generally subtle in DRESS.

A specific drug hypersensitivity is responsible for DRESS reaction. However, unlike TEN, disturbances in the drug detoxication pathway do not take place in the epidermis, but rather in other organs including the liver [136]. The impaired ability to detoxify reactive drug metabolites mainly activates a T-cell response [136]. The most common histopathological finding consists of a dense superficial perivascular lymphocytic infiltrate, associated with spongiotic or lichenoid changes, and a variable degree of edema. It has been reported that IL-1 cluster polymorphism and haplotypes, as well as the IL-10-592 A allele are associated with DRESS [137].

8.9. Systemic Lupus Erythematosus

Some rare clinical presentations of systemic lupus erythematosus (SLE) resemble SJS or TEN [138, 139]. SLE is essentially a vasculitis involving the skin and any other organ. Skin lesions are not constant or regular. Histopathology and immunopathology help distinguishing SLE from SJS and TEN. The distinct features of SLE are the superficial interface and peripilar distribution of a dense lymphoid infiltrate, intradermal deposits of glycosaminoglycans and subepidermal deposits of immunoglobulins and complement.

Chapter 9

Drug Impact

In the vast majority of TEN cases, there is a causative recent drug ingestion. A large body of evidence suggests that TEN is a SCAR resulting from a specific patch in drug metabolism generating cytotoxic compounds [94, 140]. Bioactivation of the drug and the genetic variations in genes associated with drug metabolism have been implicated in the pathogenesis of SJS, TEN and other SCAR [141-143]. More than a hundred different drugs are recognized to cause TEN, but only a minority of them account for the vast majority of cases. These offending drugs are mainly represented by antibacterial sulfonamides (co-trimoxazole), aromatic anticonvulsants (phenol-barbital, phenytoin and carbamazepine), non-steroidal anti-inflammatory agents (phenylbutazone, oxyphenbutazone, isoxicam, piroxicam, Cox-2-inhibitors), allopurinol and a series of antibiotics as well [144-147]. Among more recently introduced drugs, a strong association is documented for nevirapine (a non-nucleoside anti-retroviral agent) [148, 149], lamotrigine (an anticonvulsant), sertaline (a selective serotonin re-uptake inhibitor), panto-prazole (a proton pump inhibitor) and tramadol (an analgesic) [6, 150]. Risks are generally present during the initial 3 weeks of drug intake, and largely confined to the first 8 weeks of treatment. The total number of cases related to an individual drug clearly depends on two factors: (a) the level of risk inherent to that agent and (b) the number of patients receiving the drug.

Although ADR is the only recognized cause of TEN, some other clinical risk factors for the development of the disease were identified in the past. Among them, bacterial infections, some vaccinations [151], allogeneic bone marrow and stem cell transplantations [109, 152], SLE [138, 139, 153, 154], radiation therapy [155] and some oncologic diseases as well [156, 157].

However, as these conditions often require multi-drug treatments at risk of adverse reactions, it proves to be difficult to distinguish whether TEN is induced by the drugs or if the primary disease represents a risk factor for TEN. It is possible that these specific conditions alter the immune system, producing ADR different from those affecting the normal population.

There is no reliable test to establish the link between a single given case and a specific drug. The usefulness and the safety of in vivo skin tests remain to be established. The determination of the offending drug relies on clinical presumption mainly based on the timing of the reaction. In the most important patient series, a mean time of 14 days from initial drug administration to the onset of TEN was generally noted for all implicated drugs.

AIDS patients are recognized to be at risk for TEN [158, 159]. At least, three factors explain this feature: (a) the large number of drugs administered, (b) the altered immune system function, and (c) the possible abnormal patterns of production and/or detoxication of drug metabolites. In addition, HIV-1 is present in TEN blister fluid [160], and molecular interactions have been demonstrated in vitro between HIV and human keratinocytes [161]. Moreover, severe cutaneous ADR including TEN are associated with specific anti-HIV medications [162, 163]. By contrast, there is no association between TEN and other viral infections including human *Herpes virus*, *Cytomegalovirus* and *Parvovirus* B19 [164].

The pathomechanisms involved in drug rashes are diverse. Lesions exhibit varied histopathological presentations and clinical aspects, evolutions and outcomes.

Some clinicians consider a cluster of ADR as manifestations of a broad spectrum of related diseases, while others contend they are separate, distinct entities. The severe ADR encompass TEN, SJS, AGEP and DRESS. Based on clinical observations, TEN and SJS seem to be part of a continuum of the same pathological process.

Chapter 10

Pharmacogenetics

Although the pathogenic mechanism of SJS and TEN is not fully understood, current pharmacogenomic studies have demonstrated a correlation of HLA genes with drug-induced SJS and TEN [165-169]. Accordingly, a genetic background involving the major histocompatibility complex (MHC) possibly contributes to drug reactions including the TEN pathobiology because MHC plays a role in the control of the immune response to drugs [170].

Drugs and their metabolites are small chemicals which unlikely trigger an immune reaction by themselves. A hapten hypothesis was offered to explain drug reactions. Specific antigenic drug metabolites possibly bind covalently to some intracellular epitope peptides. In vitro investigations reported that some reactive drug metabolites interact covalently with cellular macromolecules in normal human keratinocytes [171]. The adducts potentially create toxic compounds or neoantigens recognized by the immune system. They commonly accumulate to high levels over 7-14 days under drug intake. This represents the time commonly preceding the cutaneous toxic reaction and the cell demise. The toxicity threshold of these adducts is expected to vary among individuals, possibly as a function of detoxication ability and likely corresponds to a primary determinant for developing a drug reaction. After cellular processing, some of these adducts form endogenous antigens presented on the keratinocytes surface with MHC class I molecules, resulting in a HLA-restricted CD8+ CTL recognition and activation.

Another hypothesis relies on the p-i concept dealing with the direct noncovalent pharmacological interactions of drugs with MHC molecules [172, 173]. Some studies favor the p-i concept in SJS and TEN [174]. The noncovalent interactions of drugs, such as carbamazepine or its metabolites,

HLA-B-bound peptides, HLA-B molecules of antigen-presenting keratinocytes and TCR would trigger the drug hypersensitivity [174]. In sum, both the hapten and p-i hypotheses suggest that drug-induced SJS and TEN involve the interaction of specific MHC class I molecules, T-cell receptors, and drug-modified antigens [175].

With respect to the drugs inducing TEN, significant associations were found for HLA-A29 plus HLA-B12 and HLA-B12 plus HLA-DR7 in sulfonamide-related TEN Caucasian patients. By contrast, oxicam-related TEN cases were linked to HLA-A2 and HLA-B12 [176]. In Taiwanese patients, a strong association was shown between both the antigen HLA-B* 1502 and B* 5801, and SSJ and TEN induced by carbamazepine [177] and allopurinol [178], respectively. Similarly, HLA-A* 0206 was strongly associated with SJS and TEN with ocular complications in Japanese patients [179]. Because these findings were not confirmed in Caucasian patients, the genetic markers for SJS and TEN do not appear to be universal, and ethnicity seems to be of prime importance [180-183]. However, the high sensitivity/specificity of some HLA markers provides a likely basis for developing tests identifying individuals at risk for SJS and TEN, in any given ethnic group [169].

In addition to the involvement of the MHC system, specific extrathymic education and functions of the T lymphocytes (e.g. following infection) or specific intrathymic selections in the TCR repertoire can also change the T lymphocyte reaction and cause SJS or TEN [184]. Moreover, variations in other non-HLA genes such as the Toll-like receptor 3 gene polymorphisms could be associated with SJS and TEN [185].

Chapter 11

Lymphocytic Impact

Various ADR are associated with drug-specific CTL and NK involvement [186-189]. With the identification of specific HLA alleles as predisposing factors to the ADR, both SJS and TEN correspond to severe hypersensitivity reactions. CTL and NK cells are activated and, subsequently, they carry out cell immune reactions directed at keratinocytes in a MHC I-restricted way [190].

Upon activation of these immunocytes, various cytotoxic signals, including granulysin, perforin/granzyme B, FasR/FasL, cytokines and chemokines are launched, and they mediate the disseminated keratinocyte death in skin lesions.

TEN appears to fit into a general pattern of cutaneous ADR which show drug MHC class 1 restriction and specific T-cell drug activation. CTL and their subpopulations are associated with TEN. Immunohistochemistry discloses a CD8+ CTL predominance in the epidermis, and CD4+ T cells in the dermis. Th17 have been reported to be involved in TEN [191]. Few, if any, B lymphocytes are present.

Some authors suggested that T cells were responsible for epidermal necrosis in SJS and TEN. Keratinocyte alteration was reported to be induced by perforins and other cytokines such as TNF in part released by CTL. It has not been clarified whether CTL are present in great enough number to induce direct necrosis in the epidermis, or whether they release diffusible cytokines that initiate apoptosis.

11.1. Granulysin

Granulysin is a multifunctional protein present in human CTL and NK cells, exhibiting broad cytolytic activities against a variety of targets. This compound serves as a key agent responsible for the disseminated keratinocyte death in SJS and TEN [192]. Genome-wide gene expression profiling and immuno-histochemistry reveals that granulysin is highly expressed in blister cells of affected individuals. Experimental evidence from human epidermal keratinocytes indicates that CD8 + CTL and NK cells induce cell death through releasing granulysin. Moreover, granulysin depletion significantly reduces apoptosis of keratinocytes triggered by blister fluids from SJS and TEN patients. Such findings support a functional involvement of CTL and NK cells in the pathogenesis of SJS and TEN. Furthermore, they highlight a cytotoxic mechanism that does not require direct cell contacts.

Of note, serum levels of granulysin are markedly increased and correlated with the severity of GVHR [193] mimicking SJS and TEN.

11.2. Perforin / Granzyme B

Another hypothetic mechanism underlying the cytotoxicity in SJS and TEN involves perforin and granzyme B. Both compounds represent two cytolytic proteins released by activated CTL and NK cells. Increasing levels of perforin, granzyme B, and other toxins, appear to be correlated with disease severity of drug hypersensitivity from mild maculo-papular rashes to severe TEN [42]. In addition, the inhibition of perforin/granzyme B expression attenuates the cytotoxic effect of TEN blister lymphocytes toward keratinocytes, whereas neutralization of FasR/FasL signalling by an anti-Fas monoclonal antibody fails to block cell lysis [194].

Exocytosis of cytotoxic components is one of the most potent cell death mechanisms employed by activated CTL and NK cells. Upon lymphocyte recognition of target cells, toxins to cytoplasmic granule are secreted and together induce apoptosis of the target cells [195]. They are represented predominantly by perforin, a membrane-disrupting protein and by a family of structurally related serine proteases (granzymes) with various substrate specificities. Perforin is present as a thin “key-shaped” molecule, and it is composed of multiple domains, among which a carboxy-terminal C2 domain mediates initial, Ca^{2+}-dependent membrane binding [196, 197].

Perforin usually synergizes with granzymes to carry out cytotoxicity. Granzyme B induces DNA fragmentation and different death pathways [198]. Perforin likely creates pores within the cell membranes allowing granzyme B to diffuse into the target cell and to trigger its killing activity [199]. However, numerous lines of evidence indicate that granzyme B enters the target cells independently of perforin, through receptor-mediated endocytosis or macropinocytosis. It is rapidly internalized into endosomes-like vesicles. Subsequently, perforin alters endosomal trafficking in the target cell through a process known as endosomolysis, thereby allowing the release of granzyme B into the cytosol [200, 201]. The molecular mechanisms by which perforin enables granzyme B to escape the endosomal compartment into the cytosol are not clearly established. In addition, a noteworthy amount of perforin is not present in the endosome or cytoplasm of target cells. Perforin permeabilizes the plasma membrane and possibly potentiates the uptake of granzyme into an endolytic compartment [202]. A key role in membranolytic properties of perforin facilitates granzyme B to exit to the cytosol, where it reaches access to its substrates.

In the cytosol, granzyme B induces cell death through the activation of caspase-dependent and –independent pathways. Specifically, granzyme B directly cleaves and activates the caspases. These latter compounds represent a large family of endogenous cytosolic proteases acting in a cascade to dismantle the cell. Moreover, granzyme B triggers caspase activation indirectly by processing a pro-apoptotic protein Bid into an active form. After translocation of the activated Bid to the mitochondriae, it interacts with other pro-apoptotic proteins, such as Bax and Bak to induce mitochondrial outer-membrane permeabilization (MOMP) [203]. Subsequently, Bid-mediated mitochondrial damage results in the leakage of pro-apoptotic mitochondrial mediators including cytochrome C (Cyt C), Smac/Diablo and Omi/HtrA2, into the cyotosol to increase the downstream caspase activation [204].

Granzyme B further acts on mitochondriae for inducing caspase-independent cell death through ROS generation [205]. In addition, granzyme B directly cleaves nuclear lamins, a type of intermediate filaments that mediates the structural function and transcriptional regulation in the cell nucleus, as CTL induce apoptosis during caspase blockade. This finding provides additional insight into the role of granzyme B in caspase-independent death pathways. Taken together, granzyme B elicits its killing ability through various pathways that maximize the effectiveness in granule-mediated cell death.

Chapter 12

Monocyte-Macrophage and Mesenchymal Cell Impact

Monocyte-macrophages are present in TEN where they express IL-12 and IFN-γ [206, 207]. Immunohistochemistry reveals their positivity for Mac 387, CD14, CD68, myeloperoxidase and lyzozyme [36, 93]. They are located along the dermo-epidermal junction and haphazardly dispersed in both the dermis and epidermis. By contrast, these cells are rare in partial thickness thermal burns (PTTB) [93]. The Mac 387+ macrophage density is significantly superior to the CD45RO+ lymphocytes [93].

The monocyte-macrophage lineage encompasses Factor XIIIa+ DD (Figure 4). They are numerous and plump in the superficial dermis of most TEN cases [96, 97]. By contrast, the Factor XIIIa+ DD population appears unaffected in PTTB. Of note, in TEN, the CD34+ DD remain tiny and rare. By contrast, versican fills up most dermal cells in TEN. They appear plump compared to those in PTTB. In each condition, they are evenly distributed in the superficial dermis.

Gelatinases are involved in TEN [208]. The MMP2 and MMP9 play an important role in epidermal detachment, inflammation and reepithelialization. A high amount of MMP2 was found in TEN blister fluid with the continual presence of a significantly larger proportion of its activated forms [208]. The two gelatinases are synthesized and released by distinct cell types. MMP2 is mainly produced by mesenchymal cells, while MMP9 originates from inflammatory cells and keratinocytes. Both are secreted in the form of latent zymogens which need to undergo proteolytic and autocatalytic activation.

Their expression is under the control of several cytokines, including TNF (Figure 6).

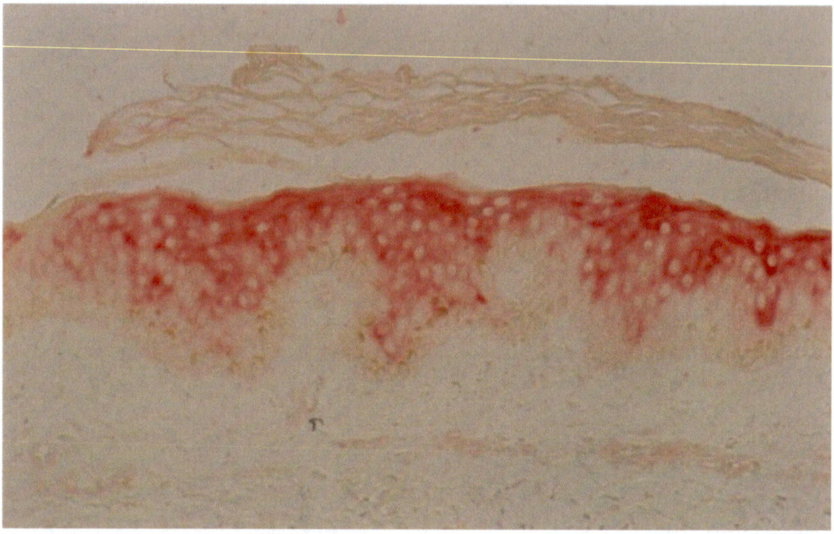

a

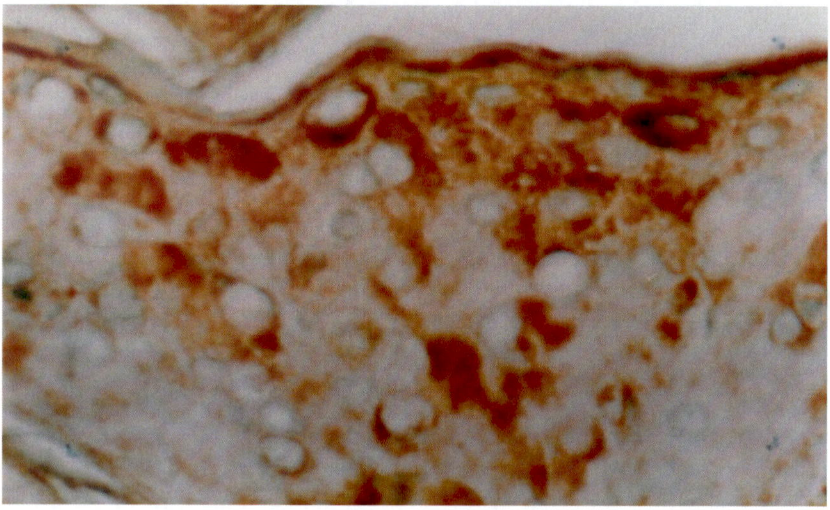

b

Figure 6. TNF immunoreactivity in TEN epidermis. a - prominent immunoreactivity in the upper epidermis. b - uneven immunoreactivity among keratinocytes.

Chapter 13

Keratinocyte Pathobiology and Demise

13.1. Oxidative Stress

The cytosolic glutathione-S-transferase (GST) family represents phase II detoxication enzymes. Specifically, a GST catalyzes the conjugation of reduced glutathione (GSH) to a variety of endogenous and exogenous electrophilic compounds following activation of GSH sulfhydryl groups. The isoenzyme GST-π is the most abundant form present in keratinocytes, and it plays a key role in the detoxication of electrophilic compounds [209]. GST-π is overexpressed in TEN keratinocytes compared to other cutaneous ADR and bullous pemphigoid [210]. Oxidative stress is one of the major inducers of GST-π expression. It is probably involved in TEN epidermal destruction through reactive oxygen species (ROS) production by electrophilic xenobiotics [211].

ROS act as intracellular chemical second messengers, and they increase gene transcription of inflammatory cytokines. Such a pathway follows transient activation by phosphorylation or allosteric modifications of redox-sensitive nuclear transcription factors such as NF-κB, AP-1 or USF43 [212]. ROS induce IL-6, IL-8 and TNF productions in keratinocytes [213, 214]. In addition, ROS directly damage some cell components including fatty acid esters of phospholipids, thus altering the membrane semi-permeability. By destabilizing membrane phosphoinositides, ROS-induced lipid peroxidation initiates the apoptotic signal cascades through the mobilization of Ca^{2+} from the endoplasmic reticulum and the activation of protein kinase C [207]. Any increase in Ca^{2+} cytosol represents an early threat in TEN keratinocytes.

GSH is a major detoxifying antioxidant for drug reactive metabolites in ADR. It directly scavenges various ROS and serves as a substrate for GST-π and the glutathione peroxidase enzyme. Human keratinocytes are resistant to toxic drugs such as sulfamethoxazole unless GSH is depleted, whereupon the cells become susceptible to the cytotoxic effects. This is of particular importance in HIV-infected patients who combine both low systemic and intracellular GSH levels [215], and an increased risk of TEN [74].

13.2. Calprotectin and Calcium

Under Ca^{2+} regulation, the S100 A8 and S100 A9 proteins form an heterotetramere S100 A8 / S100 A9 called calprotectin (L1 protein) [216]. This compound is strongly expressed in keratinocytes during TEN (Figure 7), even early in the TEN progression well before any sign of epidermal destruction [217].

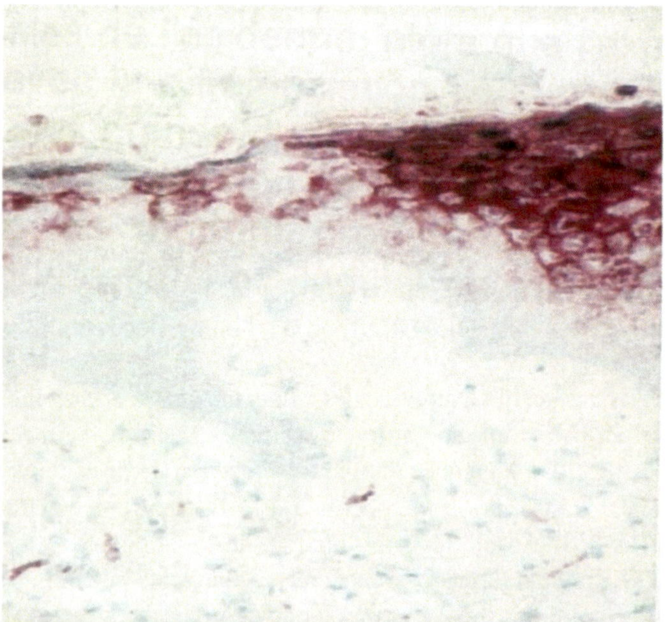

Figure 7. Focal calprotectin accumulation in TEN epidermis.

An increase in intracellular Ca^{2+} of keratinocytes is therefore an early phenomenon [217]. Such a process possibly results from (a) Ca^{2+} income from the intercellular compartment and/or (b) Ca^{2+} release from the endoplasmic reticulum corresponding to a major Ca^{2+} storing organelle, such as the Golgi apparatus and mitochondriae.

The intrusion of extracellular Ca^{2+} into cells is possible through ionic channels present in the plasmic membrane. Such structures are voltage-dependent in depolarisable cells, or voltage-independent in non-depolarisable cells. In the latter type, their function is modulated by light, mechanical stress, temperature, pH, osmolarity and any metabolic stress [218, 219].

The irregular intracellular Ca^{2+} concentrations are kept at a low level by the action of Ca^{2+}- ATPase pumps present in the plasmic membrane and the endoplasmic reticulum where they correspond to sarco-endoplasmic reticulum C^{2+}- ATPase (SERCA). These SERCA help collecting Ca^{2+} inside the endoplasmic reticulum. The Ca^{2+}- ATPases are activated by increased Ca^{2+} concentrations in the cell and by signal cascades. Any increase in cellular cytosolic Ca^{2+} amount leads to cell death by apoptosis or oncosis [220, 221].

Calprotectin is present in Mac 387+ keratinocytes in all cases of TEN irrespective of the histopathologic grade [93]. The cytoplasmic staining is focal or diffuse throughout the epidermis layers, even when the dermal inflammatory infiltrate is scarce. The uneven to strong Mac 387+ immunolabeling of keratinocytes present in all biopsies of TEN-altered skin [36, 37] indicates a cytosol load in Ca^{2+}. Calprotectin is expressed mainly in suprabasal layers of TEN epidermis, with more discrete involvement of basal keratinocytes. Most samples from apparently uninvolved skin in TEN patients express calprotectin in a patchy pattern inside the epidermis, at sites where inflammatory cells remain scanty or absent.

In PTTB, all keratinocytes show an intense Mac 387 labeling suggesting an imbalance in intracellular Ca^{2+} concentration [130].

13.3. Fas Ligand Track

FasR and FasL appear to play prominent roles in the TEN process [222]. In vitro functional studies have demonstrated that keratinocytes in TEN patients express lytically active CD95L [223, 224]. FasR is a transmembrane protein, belonging to the death receptor (DR) family which is part of the TNF receptor superfamily. FasR ligation occurs with its cognate ligand, FasL, which also corresponds to a TNF-related transmembrane molecule. FasL is expressed in a far more limited way than FasR. It allows the engagement of receptor and subsequent transduction of the apoptotic signal. Upon activation, a complex of proteins termed death-inducing signalling complex (DISC) forms and associates with activated FasR. Such protein complex encompasses the adaptor, FasR-associated death domain (FADD) protein, and procaspase-8 corresponding to a pro-apoptotic protease.

FasR/FasL interaction modulates keratinocyte apoptosis in SJS and TEN, and is of paramount importance for CTL-mediated lysis in vitro. The physiopathologic involvement of FasR and FasL on epidermal keratinocytes of TEN patients depends on increased expressions of both soluble FasL (sFasL) and epidermal FasL [225, 226]. The sFasL detected in TEN serum is derived from cleavage of the membrane-bound FasL (mFasL) present on keratinocytes. Moreover, cell death is abolished by FasL-blocking antibodies. Such findings imply the ligation of FasL expressed by TEN keratinocytes with FasR on adjacent keratinocytes as a critical step in the disease pathogenesis. However, keratinocyte FasL is primarily located inside the cytoplasm in vivo, and unable to induce apoptosis [227]. This process is further challenged by the absence of membrane-bound FasL expression on TEN keratinocytes. Increased levels of sFasL are however detected in SJS and TEN [223]. An noteworthy alterative source of serum sFasL was suggested in both SJS and TEN as sFasL levels increase significantly when peripheral blood mononuclear cells from TEN patients are cultured with the offending drug. Although FasR-FasL interactions are involved in the SJS and TEN keratinocyte death, controversy remains as to whether elevated level of sFasL in TEN serum results from cleavage of mFasL from epidermal keratinocytes or blood mononuclear cells, as well as whether TEN keratinocytes express lytically active FasL.

In addition to the regulation of apoptosis, FasR-FasL interaction plays a prominent role in the activation of NF-κB [228] and the induction of an inflammatory response [229]. These distinct effects of FasL possibly result from the functional differences in its membrane-anchored and soluble forms. Under certain circumstances, sFasL even antagonizes the effects of mFasL [230]. These diverse activities suggest that the pathogenic role of epidermal FasR expression in SJS and TEN is likely different from that of elevated sFasL detected in the serum.

13.4. Epidermal Cell Kinetics

Epidermal stem cells (ESC), transient amplifier cells (TAC) and post-mitotic cells (PMC) are present in the deep epidermal layers. The basal layer of the normal adult interfollicular epidermis contains a few ESC (0.01%), whereas TAC (40%) and PMC (50%) are more abundant. ESC represents epidermal progenitor cells exhibiting both high potential for proliferation and almost unlimited capacity for self-renewal. However, in regular conditions, they are characterized by a low rate of cell proliferation. Hence, they remain labeled for long periods of time after being exposed to tritiated thymidine (^{3}H-TdR) or bromodeoxyuridine (BrdU). These proliferation markers are retained for about one year in ESC, demonstrating these ESC quiescences. Although in vivo ESC do not commonly divide, they do so quickly both in response to specific threats and in cell culture.

ESC daughter cells corresponding to TAC undergo terminal maturation/ differentiation after dividing 3-5 times on average before leaving the basal layer. Their potential for differentiation is more restricted than that of ESC. The next step in TAC differentiation produces PMC, some of which remain attached to the basement membrane, but no longer divide. They are indeed engaged in the G0 phase of the cell cycle. Most of them start both their maturation and migration processes, moving outwards from the basement membrane. In some instance, they possibly form verrucous hyperplasias [231].

On average, ESC produce one ESC and one non-ESC, although two daughters ESC or non-ESC are possibly produced, depending on the physiologic needs of the tissue. In addition, they are vital for maintaining the global pools of ESC, TAC and PMC. It is assumed that depending on the plane of the mitosis orientation one or both daughter cells stay anchored to the basement membrane and therefore they are not immediately involved in the differentiation process.

A one-way progression from ESC to TAC represents an inadequate concept. In certain circumstances, there is evidence showing TAC being transformed into ESC. Therefore, the real role of ESC and TAC in the differentiation process remains to be established. It is yet uncertain when their role is acquired in gene functions, and what factors or markers are carried by differentiating or de-differentiating cells.

In the epidermis of the scalp, foreskin and breast, ESC are located over the tip of the dermal papillae, while they are located at the tip of the rete ridges on the palms and soles. Since ESC are located in the central part of each proliferative epidermal unit (PEU) in the basal layer or in the bulge region of the hair follicles, they are located in a special niche protected from most environmental damages.

13.5. Stem Cell Involvement

The epidermal TAC population is a major target in TEN. The risk is indeed higher in the rapidly-renewing epidermis. By contrast, ESC, which are long-term residents, remain relatively quiescent. A diversity of stem cells have been identified and two major groups are distinguished, namely the embryonic fetal stem cells and the adult stem cells. Embryonic stem cells are the most potent cells. They are capable of unlimited growth and are pluripotent, able to differentiate to any type of human tissues. By contrast, post-natal (somatic) stem cells have a limited capacity for self-renewal and they are multipotent only generating differential lineages corresponding to the tissue from which they are derived [232].

Distinct stem cell populations exist in different compartments within the skin. The ESC correspond to hair follicle bulge epithelial stem cells and stem cells in the interfollicular epidermis and sebaceous glands. In addition, bulge melanocyte stem cells and neural crest-derived stem cells have been identified in the bulge region of the human hair follicles. Mesenchymal stem cells are present in the dermis and adipose tissue.

The epidermis altered by severe damage possibly regenerates from the bulge ESC. This is likely the case in TEN. The ESC present in the bulge and interfollicular epidermis are potentially interconvertible, but under regular conditions they only differentiate a more restricted progeny.

The ESC involvement potentially influence the TEN evolution. ESC are capable of reproducing themselves in an undifferentiated state for prolonged and indeterminate periods of time. Otherwise, they differentiate themselves, and transform into more than one single type of cell with defined functions [233, 234]. In sum, the main ESC characteristics are (a) pluri- or multipotency (the ability to differentiate into different cell types), (b) plasticity (the ability to generate tissue types other than the tissue of origin), (c) quiescence (low rate of cell renewal) and (d) high proliferative potential (boosted division rate when exposed to appropriate stimuli). Such ESC are found in embryos (embryonic ESC) and in postnatal life (somatic ESC) in various tissues such as skin, bone marrow, and liver.

Two observations should be highlighted regarding TEN evolution. First, the keratinocyte repair after TEN is frequently a swift procedure contrasting with other epidermal necroses including burns and fixed drug eruptions. Second, during repair following TEN, multiple melanocytic nevi have been reported to develop [235, 236]. It is possible that the rapid epidermal recovery in the usual phase of TEN recovery results from the ESC preservation during the damaging phase. In rare instances, the healing process appears to be blocked [237, 238]. This might reflect an unusual ESC deficiency either due to the spontaneous progress of the disease or to vigorous debridement performed in the management.

In the eyes, direct damages of the corneal limbal stem cells with the loss of palisades of Vogts in the acute stage of SJS and TEN, possibly lead to a pathological stage termed limbal stem cell deficiency (SCD). Chronic blink-related microtrauma and the abnormal tear film concern to the limbal stem cells attrition, accentuating the limbal SCD. In absence of limbal epithelial stem cells, the corneal epithelium does not regenerate and the cornea is progressively invaded and covered by the surrounding conjunctival epithelium ("conjunctivalization"), as well as by an extensive fibrovascular scar, causing severe visual loss.

Ocular surface disruption occasionally develops early, as a consequence of severe inflammation in the acute stage of SJS and TEN, or manifests at a later stage, a few years after the onset of the disease. Destruction of the limbus during the acute phase is at risk of SCD, but leaves enough TAC to maintain a normal corneal epithelium for some time after the disease onset. This could explain the evolution from peripheral or localized surface failure to complete surface failure over several years in some patients.

If the reserve of limbal epithelial stem cells is preserved, repeat microtrauma to the ocular surface commonly lead to hyperproliferation-induced squamous metaplasia, generating corneal pannus similar to superior limbus keratoconjunctivitis.

13.6. Hair Follicle Privilege

Hair follicles apparently remain unaffected by SJS and TEN. Such seemingly hair follicle privilege (HFP) evokes the concept of immune privilege [239]. The term immune privilege was primarily coined in relation to tissue transplant survival in the eye (e.g., corneal allograft) and the brain.

Indeed, such transplanted tissues survive longer than anticipated. Originally, the notion of immune privilege illustrated that a given tissue environment hosting an allotransplant awarded the transplanted cells a relative protection from rejection by the host immune system.

Hair follicles are chiefly characterized by an absent or minimal level of MHC class I antigens. This pattern is complemented by a number of factors, including local production of potent immunosuppressive agents, dysfunction of professional antigen-presenting cells and inhibition of NK cell activities [239]. In the hair bulb, HFP is obvious during the anagen stage of hair cycling. In addition, the noncycling bulge area of human hair follicles enjoy some relative stable immune privilege.

Immune HFP is established and maintained by several possible ways including:

a) Downregulation or absence of MHC class I expression, which sequesters antigens in tissue sites and hinders their presentation to CD8+ CTL exhibiting a matching T-cell receptor.
b) Local production of potent immunosuppressors, such as TGF-β, IL-10 and α-MSH.
c) Functional impairment of antigen-presenting cells, occasionally by downregulating the MHC class II expression.
d) Establishment of extracellular matrix barriers to hinder immune cell trafficking.
e) Expression of unusual MHC class I molecules including the MHC class Ib molecules HLA-G.
f) Expression of FasL to delete autoreactive, Fas-expressing T-cell mechanisms.

In addition to these mechanisms of immune privilege maintenance, other processes and factors could contribute to the generation of an immune privilege environment [226]. The hair follicle stem cells could be involved [240].

There is one pathology comparison that merits some attention. It concerns the respective involvement of the epidermis and hair follicles in SJS and TEN, and the alopecia conditions corresponding to focal and generalized alopecia areata. These processes are accompanied by discrete to moderate inflammatory cell infiltrates. They distinctly correspond to apoptotic-necrotic destruction of the epidermis and hairs, respectively. In these conditions, both TAC and PMC are affected, but ESC and follicular stem cells appear commonly preserved.

Could SJS and TEN correspond to a seemingly "catagen phase" in the epidermis?

13.7. Cytokines and Chemokines in TEN Epidermal Demise

Several mechanisms of cell apoptosis induction act independently of the DR pathways. These processes act via mitochondrial damage resulting from perturbations in the balance of proapoptotic and antiapoptotic Bcl-2 proteins, e.g. from protein kinase (PK) B, p53 and granzyme activity, and activation of the ceramide pathway. Granzymes are serine proteinases that are components of CTL and NK granules. They induce apoptosis after perforin expressed by activated CTL, punches a hole in the cell membrane. Such event results from caspases by cleaving Bid, thus directly affecting the mitochondrial permeability pores, and activating caspases or noncaspase-dependent pathways. The most abundant, and most potent, in terms of apoptosis, is granzyme B which is abundant in TEN blister fluid [44].

The TNF-R1 apoptotic pathway (TNF-R1-associated death domain protein, Fas-associated death domain protein-caspase 8) can be functional in keratinocytes [241]. TNF upregulates FasR and FasL [242]. The proapoptotic TNF-R1 pathway could represent a cause of apoptosis in TEN. However, the TNF-R1-caspase pathway is usually nonoperative in normal keratinocytes. TNF-R1 signals not only to caspases, but also to NF-κB, which is generally accepted to be associated with an antiapoptotic phenotype [243]. A series of IL cytokines are activated (Figure 8).

There is a potential link of TNF to extensive apoptosis/necrosis in TEN (Fig. 8). This potent cytokine induces a variety of effects including cell apoptosis, cell activation, differentiation, and specific facets of inflammatory processes [36, 244]. TNF binding to its cell surface receptor triggers apoptosis through DISC-mediated activation of caspase cascade and mitochondrial changes. This process leads to a series of cytotoxic processes, including generation of ROS and damage to DNA by endonucleases. In addition to the apoptosis induction, the pathogenesis of SJS and TEN is partly contributed by TNF effects on inflammatory response. TNF appears to be central to the changes in the vascular endothelial permeability and to the interaction between leukocytes and the vascular endothelium [245]. In coordination with the expression of specific cell adhesion molecules, TNF recruits different populations of immunocytes [246], which fits the finding that the faint lymphoid infiltrate remains a key histopathological feature of SJS and TEN (Figure 9).

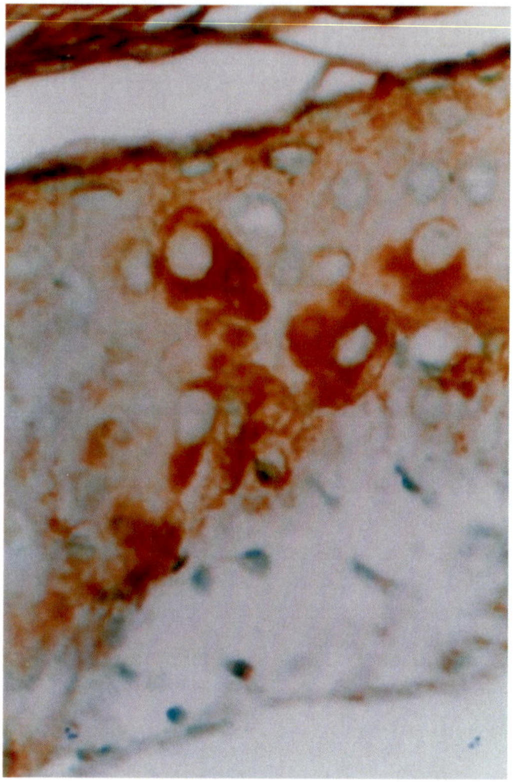

Figure 8. IL-6 immunoreactivity in TEN epidermis.

Another key cytokine playing a key role in SJS and TEN is interferon (IFN)-γ [247]. Although not transmitting apoptotic signal through a dedicated DR, IFN-γ orchestrates cytotoxic activities, to some extent, by induction of ROS. Such a mechanism connects the involvement of IFN-γ in SJS and TEN with TNF and FasL [224]. Moreover, the apoptotic effects of IFN-γ result from the transcriptional regulation of a variety of key genes for apoptosis, such as TNF receptor, FasR/FasL, caspase-1, -4, and -8. More strikingly, IFN-γ promotes antigen presentation and thus stimulate the cell-mediated immunity by upregulating MHC molecules [248], further supporting a pathogenic role in SJS and TEN.

Other than TNF and IFN-γ, numerous other cytokines and chemokines, as well as receptors responsible for the trafficking, proliferation, and activation of T-cells and other immune cells appear to be elevated in the skin lesions (Figure 8), blister fluids, blister cells, blood mononuclear cells and plasma of SJS and TEN patients. These include IL-2, IL-5, IL-6, IL-10, IL-12, IL-13, IL-15, IL-18, CCR3, CXCR3, CXCR4, and CCR10 [248, 249].

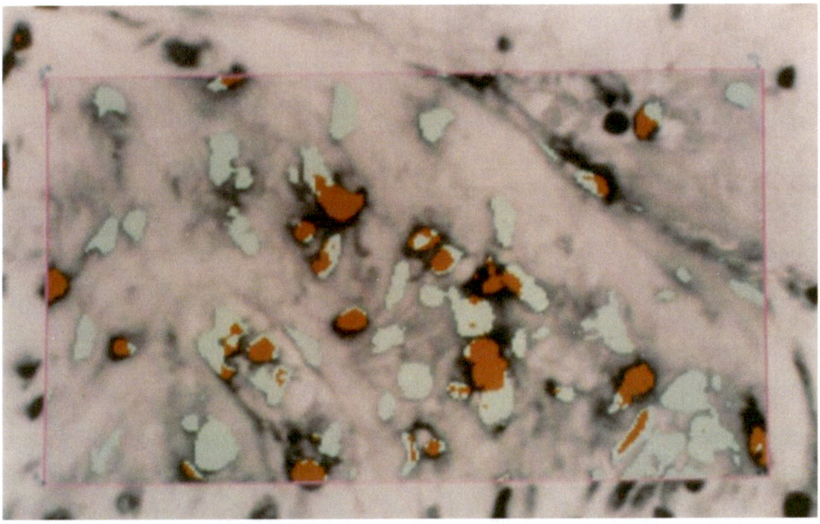

Figure 9. Image analysis processing of intraepidermal inflammatory cells in TEN: rare T lymphocytes.

Molecular and morphologic features of apoptosis are present early in SJS and TEN-involved keratinocytes. This was particularly shown by electron microscopy, as well as by the characteristic ladder pattern of DNA cleavage, and by the presence of terminal deoxynucleotidyl transferase-mediated DNA nick end labeling [250]. However, the morphologic hallmark of late apoptosis corresponding to the formation of apoptotic bodies, is not present in TEN keratinocytes. By contrast, full-thickness epidermal necrosis takes place. Hence, it is assumed that TEN pathomechanism likely combines early apoptosis and late necrosis [251]. The involvement of mitochondriae in TEN keratinocytes is a possible explanation for the simultaneous presence of these aspects of death mechanisms in TEN epidermis. Following the mitochondrial hypothesis, the TEN pathomechanism potentially involves four successive phases which intensities vary according to the degree of keratinocyte maturation [251].

The initial phase is determined by the immunogenic impact of xenobiotics. It involves the imbalance between the activation and detoxication processes in the keratinocytes. Genetic factors (slow acetylators, hyperactive peroxidase systems, ...) and/or acquired conditions (AIDS, ...) could influence this early critical phase.

The next phase corresponds to early apoptosis corresponding to a well-controlled cellular process engaging two main pathways leading to cell death [252]. The intrinsic apoptotic pathway elicits Cyt C release from mitochondriae, which leads to apoptosome formation for activating procaspase 9. The death-inducing signalling complex, another caspase-activating entity triggered by the extrinsic apoptotic pathway, stimulates proteolytic maturation of procaspase 8. Activated caspase 8 and 9, called initiator caspases, then activates the executioner caspases (caspase 3, 6 and 7) leading to the characteristic features of apoptosis. Although p53 is involved in both pathways, it appears to influence mainly the intrinsic pathway. As a transcription factor, p53 activates a number of inducible target genes that encode proteins involved in apoptosis and cell cycle regulation, while as a cytosolic protein, p53 acts in association with several members of the Bcl-2 family proteins, facilitating the mitochondrial Cyt C release.

Generation of strong electrophilic metabolites in TEN keratinocytes is expected to disrupt the electron transfer chain in the mitochondriae followed by a decline in adenosine triphosphate (ATP) production. Decreased Δym, and partial O_2 reduction are combined with ROS production. NO° metabolism is altered as well. Disrupting the electron transport chain alters the oxidative phosphorylation and abates the ATP production, thus limiting the production of GSH. Hence, any decrease in ATP production leads to impaired detoxication. The loss of Δym in mitochondriae envisions the opening of large conductance channels in the outer membrane allowing the release of Cyt C from the intermembrane location into the cytosol. Cyt C activates caspase 9 and initiates the intracellular proteolytic cascade. The process ends with apoptosis. About 1-5% of electrons transferred to O2 in the respiratory chain are derived to the superoxide anion O2-° production (O2 + e- <--> O2-°). In turn, the decrease in the coupling efficiency of electron chain transport in TEN increases the production of superoxides and ROS [253]. In TEN keratinocytes, ROS acting as second messengers likely increase gene transcription of the p55 TNF receptor and Fas pro-apoptotic systems. Indeed, increased expression of these compounds is present early in the course of TEN, both in keratinocytes and blister fluid [29, 254]. TNF probably acts as an autocrine/paracrine mediator extending the TEN epidermal destruction. In addition, TNF stimulates inducible NO synthase (iNOS) leading to the production of a large amount of NO° in TEN [255]. NO° inhibits the mitochondrial respiratory chain, enhancing intracellular $O2^{-\circ}$ production. NO° reacts with $O2^{-\circ}$ to generate high levels of the potent oxidant peroxinitrite anion $OONO^-$ (NO°+O2-°→ $ONOO^-$). The latter compound destroys Fe-S proteins and induces lipid peroxidation, thus causing irreversible damage to both mitochondriae and the intracytosolic release of Ca^{2+}. The activated CD95L+ keratinocytes are functionally able to lyse other CD95R+ keratinocytes in TEN, because CD95R is overexpressed on TEN keratinocytes [256]. Hence the CD95L / CD95R system is probably involved in early TEN apoptosis. ROS-induced lipid peroxidation makes membrane "leaky" to ions and initiates apoptotic signal cascades through Ca^{2+} mobilization from the endoplasmic reticulum and the activation of PK C [213]. Indeed, increased Ca^{2+} in the cytosol represents an early event in TEN keratinocytes. The activation of caspases, the hypercalcemia and the stimulation of pro-apoptotic cytokines such as TNF and/or CD95 lead singly or in combination to early keratinocyte apoptosis, without any intervention of inflammatory cells. Similarly, early TEN pathological features in the cornea reveal keratinocyte vacuolization without any intraepithelial lymphocyte infiltration [99, 257].

In late apoptosis, the pro-inflammatory cytokine TNF is supposed to act as an autocrine / paracrine agent acting on neighbour keratinocytes, and spreading the epidermal destruction. In addition, TNF induces the expression of the adhesion molecule ICAM-1 on keratinocytes, which corresponds to the ligand for LFA-1+ activated T lymphocytes. TNF-activated keratinocytes further produce T lymphocyte chemokines such CCL27/CTAK [258]. By their close location to the superficial capillaries, Factor XIIIa+ DD are likely activated by keratinocyte-derived cytokines, especially TNF [97]. DD are presumed to participate in TEN by acting as antigen-presenting cells and attracting inflammatory cells following secretion of appropriate cytokines [97]. Activated DD in TEN contain enlarged endoplasmic reticulum, as well as engulfed collagen fibers and mast cell granules [97]. They probably play a role in the regulation of the connective tissue remodelling that usually follows epidermal destruction.

During the late apoptosis phase, inflammatory cells accumulate the TEN epidermis. At first, they are predominantly composed of activated CD8+ CTL. They express the cutaneous lymphocytes antigen (CLA) molecules [187, 259, 260], CD25 (IL2 receptor) [49, 261], CD56 (NK cell) [187], CD69 (activation marker) [260], CD45R0 (memory T cells) [260], CD94 (NK cell receptor) [187], CD158a/CD158b (NK-cell receptor) [187], CD95L [44] and CCR10

(CTAK receptor) [258]. Functionally, they are engaged in a Tc1 pathway, producing IFN-γ and inducing overexpression of MHC class I molecules on activated keratinocytes [248, 249]. They are drug-specific, MHC class I restricted and they exhibit a perforin/granzyme-mediated cytotoxicity [262]. Further to their NK receptors, these T cells exert some functional NK cytotoxicity [187]. Thus, they are NKT-like cells, but distinct from regular CD-1d-dependent NKT cells [190].

The tissue areas where T lymphocyte are activated in TEN remain to be established. TEN peripheral lymph nodes exhibit only a discrete hyperplasia of the paracortical T cell zone with a very low Ki-67 proliferation index. Moreover, the antigen-presenting cells such as CD1a+ Langerhans' cells and Factor XIIIa+ dendritic cells are sparce in TEN lymph nodes [96]. Some cytokines including IL-15, locally induce functional NK-cell receptor expression (e.g. CD94) on T lymphocytes responding to superantigens or to alloantigens [263]. Later on, CD68+ macrophages form the most prevalent inflammatory cell population [187, 264]. They strongly interact in a mutual activation with T lymphocytes. These two activated cell populations finally lead to a late and boosted apoptotic process.

The next TEN stage is characterized by the loss of Δym leading to PT pore opening associated with osmotic disturbances in mitochondriae due to the matrix hyperosmolarity. The resulting expansion of the matrix space corresponds to organelle swelling and subsequent rupture of their outer membrane. Cells with ruptured mitochondriae are at risk of death through a slow nonapoptotic mechanism resembling necrosis [253].

In short, TEN epidermal destruction combines apoptosis at the beginning of the disease and necrosis as a later event. At each moment of the disease course, the relative proportions of the keratinocytes in early apoptosis (self-induced by the keratinocytes), in late apoptosis (induced by inflammatory cells) and in necrosis likely determine the clinical and histopathological aspect of the involved area [251].

In keratinocytes, ROS production occurs during the initial 2 hours [265], CD95 expression near the third hour, and TNF production occurs after about 24 h. The loss of Δym and caspase activation needs a period of 6-12 h [265]. The apoptotic process ensues after 24-48 h [266]. Such short intervals mean that cutaneous TEN involvement is a swift process and requires an emergency treatment.

Moreover, an immunological memory develops early after a first episode of TEN and persists for several years. This is evidenced by the rapid and generally dramatic TEN recurrence following accidental or provoked re-exposure to the offending drug [267, 268]. Provocation tests have been previously performed, but they are ethically unacceptable owing to their inherent hazards. They showed a positive result when they were performed soon after the acute onset of TEN (up to 3 months) [269], but gradually became negative as the interval from the past eruption increased.

In a global view, the DR pathways for TNF, FasL and TNF-related apoptosis-inducing ligand (TRAIL) which signal through Fas-associated death domain protein (FADD) to caspase 8 and cause apoptosis [270]. In addition, TNF can signal to NF-κB, which is antiapoptotic. The non-DR pathways work via the mitochondrial pore. Granzyme B signals through this pathway or via noncaspase-dependent pathways. TNFR-1, TRAF (TNFR-associated factor), IKK (I-kB kinase), TRADD (TNFR-1-associated death domain protein), FasR, TRAIL-R1, 2 (TRAIL receptors 1 and 2), PKB, protein G, GD3 (galactoside GD3), APAF1 (apoptotic protease activating factor).

13.8. Systemic Consequences

Common aspecific complications of TEN encompass massive daily fluid losses (up to 4 litres) through the altered epidermis in adults with epidermal necrolysis extending over 50% of TBSA, bacterial colonization of the skin initiating systemic sepsis, rises in serum amylase, lipase, creatine phosphokinase and aminotransferase. Anemia is present in most patients due to erythroblastopenia and disseminated intravascular coagulation. Various alterations in the immune response include lymphopenia due to depletion of CD4+ helper T lymphocytes, decreased chemotactic and phagocytic activity of granulocytes, depletion of serum immunoglobulins, impaired in vitro response of lymphocytes to recall antigens and decreased CTL and NK responses. In addition, acute skin failure contributes to a hypercatabolic state. Inhibition of insulin secretion and/or insulin resistance in peripheral tissues result in elevated plasma glycemia and frequent glycosuria.

Several epithelia of internal organs are occasionally involved in the TEN process, mainly the respiratory and gastrointestinal tracts, and the kidneys. Rare cases of encephalopathy, myocarditis or rhabdomyolysis potentially develop in acute SJS and TEN.

Chapter 14

Analytic Skin Biometrology

14.1. Reflectance Skin Colorimetry

Skin colors show wide interindividual differences. They depend on genetic factors (ethnicities, phototype), environmental factors (suntanning) and local cutaneous factors (scar, striae distensae, frictions). In addition, skin colors show large variations according to the body sites. Even on a small spot (± 1 cm^2) dedicated techniques commonly reveal some heterochromy.

Instrumental assessments of epiluminescence skin colors using dedicated metrological devices result in more objective, reproducible and quantitative information than visual scoring only. Epiluminescence skin colorimetry is conveniently measured instrumentally using reflectance methods. Reflectance colorimetry takes advantage of the CIEL*a*b* standardized system in the L*a*b* color space notifications. Value L* representing lightness is expressed on a scale ranging from 0 for black to 100 for white. The positive values a* and b* are expressed in the 0-100 range in two perpendicular color axes, with a* corresponding to the red hue and b* to the yellow hue [271-273].

Color differences between the target and the reference areas are calculated following a substraction (Δ) between the dual figures of the same colorimetric parameter (ΔL^*, Δa^*, Δb^*). Any positive Δ value indicates that the hue under consideration is more pronounced on the target area than that on the reference area. The overall difference in color is given by ΔE^* ab following: $\Delta E^*ab=[(\Delta L^*)^2 + (\Delta a^*)^2 + (\Delta b^*)^2]^{0.5}$.

The transformation formula $\tan^{-1}$ (b*/a*) is defined as hue and stands for redness purity [274]. Another way for expressing erythema relies on the calculation of differences between sites regarding (L*.a*)b*[1]. The difference between two measures is informative. Still another means relies on the calculation of skin colors in the three-dimensional CIE L*a*b* color space using vectorial representation. The determination of the skin color volume (SCV) appears relevant.

Few studies have been performed so far about skin colorimetry in TEN. Assessments were performed between erythematous sites covered by the epidermis. The $(L^*.a^*)b^{*-1}$ was higher on sites remaining covered by the epidermis for at least 48h compared to other sites undergoing a rapid epidermal sloughing off. Such a colorimetric procedure could therefore be used to predict a severity score of lesional skin extension for the next 48h, at least in absence of systemic involvement.

14.2. Field Melanin Mapping

In Humans, melanocytes and their melanin production are responsible for the phototype-related skin color. Two chemically distinct types of melanins are present in the skin, namely an insoluble black-brown eumelanin and an alkali soluble red-yellow phaeomelanin. The microenvironment abutted to the melanosomes enriched with these pigments is critically important. Indeed, the varied skin hues depend largely on the chemical nature, amount and distribution of melanin pigments produced in melanosomes and transferred to keratinocytes. The overall system appears organized in epidermal melanin units (EMU) corresponding to functional entities each composed of a single melanocyte and its neighbouring keratinocytes into which melanosomes are transferred. Chronic exposures to ultraviolet light (UVL) radiations provide an incentive signal to the photo-exposed EMU. As a result, most individual active melanocytes are stimulated to produce more melanin to EMU.

A discrete focal subclinical melanoderma develops on most body areas of Caucasian people over the years. Such presentation has been named faint mosaic melanoderma (FMM). This focal pattern of increased melanin pigmentation is apparently uninvolved in the development of any melanocytic tumor, either benign or malignant. By contrast, FMM appears to initiate a modified clinical presentation corresponding to melanotic hypermelanosis. In addition, according to the age of the subject, the skin phenotype, the hormonal status and the cumulative chronic UVL exposures, skin commonly develops a progressive clinically recognizable mottled melanotic presentation [275]. The aspects result from an increase in the melanin content inside keratinocytes (melanotic hypermelanosis) associated or not with melanocyte hyperplasia. The resulting mottled pigmentation is an early key manifestation of a genetically controlled skin response to sustained UVL exposure. Freckles in youths, melasma in young women and solar lentigines in older individuals are typical lesions issued from such a process.

The FMM observations require special UV lighting of the skin [273-275]. The methods particularly rely on the envision of UVA which spectrum of wavelengths spans from 320 to 400 nm [276, 277]. During the reepithelialization phase at the issue of TEN, the FMM frequently exhibits a contrasted pattern. An overall increased EMU activity is present leading to a possible hyperpigmentation.

14.3. Skin Capacitance Mapping

The electrical properties of skin are influenced by (a) its surface texture and microrelief, (b) by the water and electrolyte content in the SC, and (c) by the sweat production as well. Measuring electrical capacitance is a convenient although indirect way to appreciate any changes in these physiologic parameters [266]. The capacitance method is rooted on the permittivity of water (e = 81), which is higher than for most other molecules. Thus, the dielectric characteristics of the SC mainly depend on its water content, so that a broad range of determinations is possible. According to the location of the measurement site, sources of error and potential sources of variation in the data are encountered including sweat production, occlusion of the sweat ducts, density in vellus hairs, as well as the electrolyte content of the SC, and some artefacts from applied xenobiotics.

A recent technological advance has been made, with the design of the skin capacitance mapping/imaging (SCM) method, representing a specific type of nonoptical skin surface imaging [278-280]. This method relies on fine-tuned electrometric measurements of the skin surface properties. During the TEN progression phase, the aspect of SCM takes a darker look probably related to an altered skin barrier function. Such aspect is interpreted as a predictor for the extension of the epidermal involvement.

14.4. In Vivo Reflectance Confocal Microscopy

In vivo reflectance confocal microscopy (RCM) of the skin [281-283] is a noninvasive, high-resolution method providing in vivo imaging of the skin. RCM provides real-time recordings of cell shapes and overall structures of superficial tissues down to a depth of about 200 μm. The images are captured in horizontal planes. The observed skin tissues are not subjected to chemical fixation and staining. Thus, their native structures remain intact. Furthermore, RCM allows repeat observations of the same location. Therefore, the findings shed light on any dynamic aspect including tissue destruction, progression, and response to treatment. One of the emerging and intriguing applications of RCM is the in vivo evaluation of disease progression. The RCM advantage appears obvious in the assessment of the dynamics of treatment responses.

Corneal TEN lesions are possibly examined using RCM [284].

Part III: Management

Chapter 15

TEN Prevention

With the advances uncovering some biopathologic aspects and pharmacogenetic characteristics of SJS and TEN, a susceptibility screening could be planed as a guideline-based test before administration of certain potentially offending drugs [176-179,285-288].

Regulatory inflammatory cells could theoretically be offered to prevent TEN [289]. In fact, thymus-derived regulatory T cells cooperate with $CD11c^+$ dendritic cells to prevent life-threatening skin damage including TEN. Patients with AIDS are at increased risk of cutaneous ADR such as TEN. The low number of $CD4^+$ cells in AIDS patients is a good marker of disease progression. Prospective evaluation of risk factors for cutaneous ADR in AIDS patients revealed that high $CD8^+$ cell numbers indicated a risk of drug eruption [290]. Thymus-derived $CD4^+$ $CD25^+$ regulatory T cells can prevent severe epidermal damage induced by auto-reactive CTL. In conventional T cell differentiation, there is evidence that the thymus is necessary for maturation of most T cells, especially ab T cells. However, a rare population, termed extrathymic T cells, differentiates without the thymus. Although the character of these unconventional T cells is still unclear, the intestines and liver are the major sites of differentiation [291].

Avoiding the administration of the causative drug and any compound showing some similarities with it is primordial [292]. At present, there is no other way to prevent the extension of the lack of skin integrity in TEN.

Antishear therapy reducing friction on the skin [293] likely prevent the extension of the epidermal detachment.

Chapter 16

Prognosticators

The cutaneous and mucosal destruction in TEN is related to high incidence of water, electrolyte, protein losses and thermoregulatory disturbance. Increasing age, severe comorbidity and greater extent of skin involvement correlate with a worse prognosis [7]. The main factors involved in TEN mortality are the occurrence of sepsis at the time of hospitalization, age, and total body surface area involved. The presence of comorbidities (sepsis, renal failure, lung distress, diabetes, tuberculosis, AIDS, ...) and steroid intake are individually important although they do not represent independent variables.

It is important to follow the algorithms of imputability methods of drug causality used for ADR [294-300]. The ALDEN algorithm has recently been promoted [301] and is used in current therapeutic assessments [302].

The identification of independent risk factors for death initiated the SCORTEN (severity of illness score for TEN) determination. SCORTEN is based on seven risk factors [294-300], namely, age over 40 years, presence of malignancy, initial epidermal detachment of more than 10% of body surface, heart beat over 120/min, glycemia above 252 mg/dL (14.0 mmol/L), serum bicarbonate level less than 20 mmol/L, and serum urea level above 27 mg/dL (10 mmol/L). Hypernatremia and tuberculosis are other factors affecting the mortality [303]. Major drugs involved are listed in Table I. The SCORTEN value varies in time, and its best prediction is reached on day 3 post-admission [296]. It is generally considered as an accurate estimate of the risk of death in TEN [304]. However, some authors consider that mortality is possibly overestimated in the setting of up-to-date treatment protocols.

Table I. Drugs with a high relative risk for TEN

Aromatic anticonvulsant	Phenobarbital Phenotrine Carbamazepine Valproic acid Lamotrigine
Sulfonamide antibiotics	Sulfamethoxazole Co-trimoxazole (trimethoprim-sulfamethoxazole)
Xanthine-oxidase inhibitor	Allopurinol
Antibiotics	Aminopenicillin Cephalosporins Quinolones Tetracyclines
Nonsteroidal anti-inflammatory drugs	Oxicam Diclofenac
Pain killers	Acetaminophen Tramadol
Antiretroviral drug	Nevirapine
Others	Sertraline Tetrazepam

Conversely, others claim that respiratory involvement, and tuberculosis portend a poor prognosis that is not assessed in SCORTEN. Hence, although SCORTEN remains a useful tool predicting mortality in TEN, it should probably be further refined [299].

The extent in cell inflammation in TEN skin has been suggested to predict the clinical outcome similarly to SCORTEN. However, the value of this microscopic assessment is not an independent factor as the extent in inflammation varies according to the duration of the disease. In addition, the objective quantification of the inflammatory infiltrate is particularly difficult to perform. The major signs of differential diagnosis are listed in Table II.

An alternative rating system was proposed as the illness auxiliary score (IAS) of clinical severity. In this assessment, age appear to exert a major impact on TEN survival (Table V). In addition, HIV infection is a major factor associated with increased TEN mortality [158-163, 305].

The reported mortality of TEN ranges from 25% to 40%, which can be even higher in elderly patients and in those with large surface area of epidermal sloughing. Death often results from sepsis and metabolic disturbances resulting from the epidermal deficiency (Table III). Persistent TEN complications are common (Table IV).

Table II. Differential diagnosis

Disease	Clinical characteristics	Skin pathology
Exfoliative dermatitis	Desquamation; no mucous membrane lesions	No epidermal necrosis
SSSS	Superficial detachment; no mucous membrane lesions	Subcorneal split
AGEP	Confluent superficial pustules. Mucous membrane lesions unusual	Subcorneal pustules
Paraneoplastic pemphigus acantholysis	Subacute progression. Positive Ig deposits	Apoptotic keratinocytes Acantholysis
Generalized fixed drug eruption	Mucous membrane lesions Unusual, well-demarcated erythematous patches and erosions Previous similar reactions	Epidermal necrosis; similar to TEN
SJS	Same spectrum of disease Less extensive detachment (<10% of TBSA)	Epidermal necrosis identical to TEN
Erythema multiforme major	Typical targets Less extensive detachment (<10% of TBSA)	Interface dermatitis; no necrosis
Thermal burns	History Suggestive distribution	Mimics necrolysis
Pressure blisters	Suggestive distribution No targets or macules No mucous membrane lesions	May mimic TEN

Table III. Mortality risk related to the SCORTEN value

SCORTEN	Expected mortality rate (%)
0-1	3.2
2	12.1
3	35.3
4	58.3
5	90

Table IV. Persistent TEN complications

Tissue/Organ	Clinical sign
Skin	• Patchy hypo- and/or hyperpigmentation • Diffuse pruritus • Hypertrophic/cheloidal scarring • Eruptive melanocytic nevi • Verrucous hyperplasia
Eyes	• Dry eye syndrome • Photophobia • Ocular pain • Loss of visual acuity • Chronic conjunctivitis sicca • Tarsal conjunctiva keratinization • Conjunctival synechia • Ectropion • Entropion and trichiasis • Lid adhesion, symblepharon • Corneal neovascularization • Corneal opacification • Corneal abrasions, ulcers • Lacrymal duct scarring • Recurrent lacrymal cysts
Nails	• Dystrophy • Ridging • Streaky pigmentation of the nail bed • Growth-stunted nails
Oral cavity	• Chronic tongue ulcerations • Synechia between tongue/lips and gingiva • Xerostomy and Sjogren-like syndrome • Parotid cyst • Hypopharyngeal stenosis and dysphagia
Genital mucosae	• Vulvar adenosis • Vulvar atrophy • Chronic vulvar ulceration • Synechiae between the minor and major labia • Vestibular or introital stenosis • Vaginal dryness • Phimosis

CIAS prognosticators are listed in Table V.

Table V. Criteria of illness auxiliary score

Variables	Score value
Age 31-55 years 56-75 years >75 years TEN (involved TBSA > 30%) Presence of malignancy	 1 2 3 1 1
Expected mortality (%)	**Global score value**
4 10 21 40 63 >63	0 1 2 3 4 5

Stem cells possible involved in TEN are identified in Table VI.

Table VI. Stem cell identification markers

Stem cells	Markers
Interfollicular stem cells	CK15, CD10, CD71, p63
Infundibular stem cells	Lrg1, Sca1
Isthmus stem cells	Lrg6, MTS24
Sebaceous stem cells	Blimp1, CK5/14
Bulge stem cells	CD200, CK15, CD34 (CD24, CD71)
Neural crest derived stem cells	Nestin, Slug, Twist, Sox10
Perivascular stem cells	NG2, CD34
Adipose-derived stem cells	CD29, CD44, CD71, CD90, CD105, SH3.

Chapter 17

Supportive Care Management

17.1. General Supportive Measures

Prompt diagnosis and expeditious referral of TEN patients to a multidisciplinary teamwork in a burn center or an intensive care unit considerably helps reducing morbidity and mortality [306-310]. The patient should be oriented to an isolation room. Nursing on specialized units is clearly of paramount importance for preventing complications. Adequate nursing care, includes protection of exposed dermis and mucosal surfaces, management of electrolyte and energy intake, pain control, sedation, and detection and treatment of infections. Such commitments have to be initiated soon after admission [41]. Prompt withdrawal of the suspected causative drug and avoidance of any chemically-related drug are of paramount importance for decreasing the amount of electrophilic metabolites, and improving the prognosis [311]. It remains that there are no controlled trials assessing supportive care in TEN. Although intuitively logical, there is only limited evidence of an effect on the course of the disease.

So far, there are no in vitro rapid and reliable tests to identify the causative drug in TEN [290, 312-315]. The probability of involvement of a specific drug in TEN remains based on a series of clinical and pharmacological algorithms rather than on in vitro tests [24, 315]. Drugs sharing any chemical similarity with the initial offending compound must be discarded when possible in the management of TEN since the risk of TEN recurrence and fatal cross-reactivity is high [24, 315, 316].

The main principles of supportive therapy for TEN is similar to that used in severe burn patients. The reduction of pain at the wounded sites is important to perform. It is conveniently assessed using a visual analog pain scale in which 0 indicates no pain and 10 indicates the strongest or unbearable pain. Pain intensity should be recorded on the day of admission (before debridement), and every second day for at least 2 weeks.

During the first few days, fluids must be replaced intravenously. When possible, it is preferable to use peripheral veins at a distance from affected areas rather than central lines. The predicted volume of replacement is proportional to the area of skin erosions. However, the fluid requirements of TEN patients are two-thirds to three-fourths of those of patients with burns covering the same area.

Early TEN involvement of the respiratory tract is associated with poor prognosis, and high risk for acute respiratory failure. Early mechanical ventilation (1-4 day after hospital admission) is required for most of these patients and remains bound to a high (> 65%) mortality rate.

There is generally a good correlation between bacteria isolated from the skin and those isolated from bacterial pneumonitis. This helps to treat empirically the lung infection before complete identification of the pathogens responsible for pneumonitis. These germs generally include MRSA, *Streptococcus pneumoniae* and *Acinetobacter baumannii.* Patients with delayed pulmonary manifestations do not consistently require mechanical ventilation. However, those who need it have a poor prognosis with a 50% mortality.

Eating is commonly painful and difficult. Appropriate nutritional support is mandatory [317, 318]. Enteral nutritional support is preferable to parenteral nutrition, as it is better tolerated. It is started as soon as possible by naso-gastric route with a silicone tube to minimize the protein losses and to promote healing of the cutaneous lesions. An immune stimulating nutrition has been proposed [316]. Because of impaired glycoregulation, intravenous insulin is frequently required. Environmental temperature should be raised to 30-32°C. This reduces caloric losses through the skin and the resultant shivering and stress. Heat loss is also limited by raising the temperature of antiseptic baths to 35-38°C, and by using heat shields, infrared lamps, and a temperature-controlled air-fluidized bed. Immune modulating enteral nutrition might be considered [310].

Hyperglycemia in critically ill patients is associated with increased morbidity and mortality [319]. Patients with TEN may be physiologically stressed, in pain, and have sometimes been treated with systemic steroids.

These factors combined with hyperalimentation make hyperglycemia likely. It is noteworthy that hyperglycemia is an identified risk factor used in the SCORTEN severity scoring system in TEN. Strict control of blood glucose with an insulin sliding scale infusion should be applied [319]. There is additional evidence that insulin has an antiapoptotic action that is of some benefit in TEN patients.

17.2. Skin Supportive Measures

Two firmly established principles improve survival in the management of TEN. They correspond to early withdrawal of the offending drug and prompt referral to a burn unit. Control of the skin bacterial colonization and infection is critical in TEN management. The burn unit environment is considered as an optimal place for widespread wound management as they provide a relatively isolated and appropriate ward for TEN patients. Early transport to a burn unit or to a similarly qualified specialized center should be the standard care for TEN.

Antibiotics should be only administered in case of evidence for a specific focus of infection [14, 16, 17, 19, 23]. A prophylactic use is therefore not recommended. By contrast, care must be taken in screening for sepsis and surveillance of lines/catheters to allow prompt intervention. All patients should be bathed. Application of a broad spectrum topical antimicrobial gauze is recommended to cover the wounds and changed daily under sedation to prevent wound sepsis.

The dry crust which is part of the autologous tissue represents a biological dressing. It helps reducing effusion under the dressing and further contributes to avoid infection. The microspheres in air-fluidized beds contribute to form clumps of effusion. They bring the bacteria away and fall to the diffuser board present at the bottom of the bed. They are then desiccated by airflow and they rise again shortly afterwards, and eventually form a cycle in this way.

17.3. Eye Supportive Measures

Daily examination of the fornices must be performed by an ophthalmologist [320]. Following application of topical anesthetic, the fornices are swept by a round-typed muscle hook or scleral depressor to assess for early symblepharon. Symblepharon rings are oval-shaped with a round window cut out over the cornea. They fill the fornices and provide separation of the palpebral and bulbar conjunctiva. The largest rings are best indicated because they allow eyelid closure. In children, sedation is usually necessary for the initial placement, but the rings are generally well tolerated once in place [321]. The integrity of the corneal epithelium is maintained by bandage contact lenses, but such a procedure should be taken with caution due to the risk of infection [62].

Any mucinous, aqueous and lipidic component of the tear film is potentially affected in chronic SJS and TEN. Marked ocular surface dryness represents a common disease sequel. Prominent eyelid scarring often closes the lacrymal drainage system and renders it non-functional. If the system remains patent, occlusion by punctual plugs or cautery is used. Frequent lubrication with preservative-free artificial tear formulations (drops, gels, ointments) represents a first-line therapy. Although artificial tear formulations bring moisturization and temporary relief for patients with ocular surface disorders, they fail to provide some important components found in natural tears. By contrast, autologous serum eye drops contain a series of these components, including epidermal growth factor, vitamin A and fibronectin. In addition, they exhibit epitheliotrophic properties and help corneal wound healing. Their benefit in patients with ocular surface disorders is commonly reported, but concerns regarding infection, lack of standard protocols and cost have limited their use.

Scleral lenses completely vaults over the cornea and limbus. They are supported entirely by the sclera, and they do not touch the cornea. They protect the ocular surface from blind-related microtrauma encountered in case of tarsal conjunctival and lid margin disease [322]. They contribute to control moisture evaporation by acting as a gas-permeable protective covering for the cornea. Such scleral lenses are proposed to patient with severe chronic ocular surface lesions associated with SJS and TEN. Indeed, these conditions including dry eye symptoms, superficial punctuate keratitis, trichiasis/ districhiasis, symblepharon and visual loss are occasionally refractory to other therapies. In most of these patients, the lenses provide symptom relief and visual rehabilitation. However, they have to be applied as a continuous wear and long-term therapy, what possibly provide some ocular discomfort. Those patients with an important build up of eye debris have to remove and clean their scleral lenses several times a day. Giant papillary conjunctivitis, infectious keratitis and visible corneal edema further occur in some patients.

Chapter 18

Survival Management

Early referral to a bun center unit reduces the TEN mortality rate [323]. Similarly to a serious burn site, death of the epidermis occurs almost instantaneously at a TEN skin lesion. The cutaneous and mucosal destruction in TEN is responsible to high incidence of water, electrolyte, protein losses and thermoregulatory disturbance. Fluid loss triggers systemic reactions that can lead to a lowered heart rate. They result in physiologic and immunologic changes, and they possibly lead to kidney, lung, liver and heart failures. Thus, vital parameters of liver, lung, kidney and heart functions as well as water and electrolyte levels should be monitored routinely.

Pulmonary involvement is common in TEN [324]. The hospital environment has a low ambient air moisture, compounding any airway damage. Treatment includes nebulized saline, bronchodilators and physiotherapy. Hypoxia usually indicates involvement of respiratory epithelium and requires supplementary oxygen, or even mechanical ventilation. Supplementary oxygen is both cold and dry. Care must be taken to humidify inspired gases. In TEN patients, face-masks are not usually well tolerated. Pressure and friction associated with a face-mask increase skin loss around the nose and mouth. This applies particularly to a continuous positive airway pressure mask, an otherwise useful therapy when respiratory failure is imminent.

Respiratory failure represents a bad prognostic sign. Those individuals requiring formal ventilation are expected to be ventilator dependent for some time and there is a risk of ventilator-associated pneumonia. Early tracheostomy may be beneficial, as it allows patients to avoid or reduce sedation, and to contribute more actively to ventilation, thus reducing respiratory muscle atrophy. Patients who are able to cough and actively contribute to clearance of sputum are at reduced risk of significant chest infection.

Chapter 19

Topical Treatment

19.1. Skin

The risk of infection is common anytime during the course of TEN. In addition, the daily transcutaneous fluid loss is markedly increased, and the balance in body temperature is impaired. The wound management plays an important role in preventing sepsis spreading from the epidermal destruction. No specific gold standard approach to wound care is presently recognized for TEN. Most treatment centers use management procedures similar to those of burn care. Maintaining proper fluid balance and body temperature are primary concerns. Sterile handling of patients is required for preventing or at least decreasing the risk of nosocomial infections [325].

19.1.1. Debridement

Debridement of the wet necrotic epidermis and the protein-rich blister fluid are advocated and commonly performed [14, 17, 19, 22, 23, 326]. Indeed, the nonviable macerated TEN epidermis still adhering to the skin represents a prominent driving force responsible for sepsis. A conservative approach only removes the epidermis that is easily peeled off. A larger operative debridement removes intact blisters and any area showing a positive Nikolsky sign. The timing of the procedure is variable among different burn-TEN centers. Large debridement requires a whirlpool mechanical procedure or a sharp debridement under general anesthesia in the operating room. Still another procedure uses a high velocity saline forced through a narrow operating window (Versajet® system) [326]. Thereafter, the TEN patient benefits from daily baths using topical liquid antiseptics.

19.1.2. Wound Closure

In debridement, procedures activated in different TEN-burn centers are variable, including the timing and extent of surgical removal, as well as the approach for closing the epithelial defect by biologic or synthetic dressings. Bioactive skin substitutes consist of porcine xenografts [327], human amniotic membrane for severe acute ocular damages [56, 328-330], fresh or cryopreserved human skin allografts, collagen sheet dressings [331], as well as autologous and allogenic cultured keratinocytes [307]. Skin substitutes [332] and tissue-engineered skin constructs offer great promises [333]. In addition, transplantation of stem cells is viewed as a great advance for boosting the repair rate in severe epidermal lesions in ADR [334]. Synthetic dressings include custom-knitted nylon fabric coated or not with a layer of porcine type 1 collagen, and mechanically bonded to an ultrathin silicone membrane (Biobrane®, Suprathel®) [335-338], nanocrystalline silver dressings (Acticoat®, Aquacel®-Ag) [339-341], calcium alginate fibers [342] and hydrofiber silver dressings. Some of these dressings are expensive, some are difficult to obtain, and the evidence for their efficacy remains commonly lacking by large multicenter studies.

The moist and clean eroded surface is possibly treated with gauze dressing covered by an antiseptic ointment like silver nitrate [343], povidone-iodine (not over 20% of TBSA owing to a potential impact on thyroid function) or chlorhexidine [14, 16, 17, 19, 22, 23, 41]. Silver sulfadiazine is used only if TEN has not been induced by sulfonamides. Topical antiseptics and sulfonamides have been claimed to exert in vitro noxious effects on keratinocytes. However, in clinical practice, these treatments protect against exogenous bacterial contamination and colonization, and thus limit the local biocenosis and offer a beneficial effect on reepithelialization [344]. Painting and bathing with topical liquid antiseptics such as 0.5% silver nitrate and 0.05% chlorhexidine, is monitored by semi-quantitative bacterial samplings on several sites of TEN-altered skin every other day.

Air-fluidized beds are successfully used for treating burn patients, pressure ulcers, TEN patients and in a series of other clinical conditions. They help drying the skin surface and they avoid maceration [310]. Air fluidized beds provide a structure for patients to float on by pumping air to silicone-coated microspheres beneath a polytetrafluoroethylene sheet, and they are separated from patient by the flowing air. The adjusted temperature of air-fluidized bed helps controlling the core body temperature. It represents a great help especially for the patients lacking the epidermal coverage, and suffering large fluctuations in body temperature. However, such a care procedure is occasionally responsible for severe hypothermia [345]. It remains that both the warm microclimate and the low interface pressure reduce the pain of patients. The application of air-fluidized beds to TEN patients reduces the time to complete re-epithelialization, releases pain and the incidence of cutaneous infections. However, any air flow increases the daily skin evaporative water losses by 5 to 6 liters, thus complicating the management of fluid and electrolyte balance [310]. The low pressure provided by air-fluidized bed decreases the likelihood of capillary closure in the wound bed or at risk tissue and further increases the exchange of nutrient and oxygen, resulting in reduced secondary trauma and tissue damage as well as better wound healing status for patients.

There is evidence that any of the extrinsic wound managements does not significantly reduce the mortality in TEN patients [346]. Moreover, contrasting with burns, the TEN course remains unpredictable, evolving over two weeks on average. This necessitates grafting in several steps, involving risky handling of the patient.

Painful involvement of mucous membranes (oral, nasal and vaginal) is constant in TEN. Frequent debridements, adequate analgesia with viscous lidocaine, and repeat applications of antibacterials and antifungals are required.

In short, TEN topical treatment could be scheduled as a two step procedure. In the early phase, a controlled debridement of necrotic skin, and the use of temporary bioactive or synthetic dressings, are important. During the later re-epithelialization phase, topical antiseptics or antibiotics, overlaid with non-adherent dressings or petrolatum gauzes guarantee a favourable environment, stimulating keratinocyte proliferation and migration.

19.2. Eye

Amniotic membrane (AM) transplantation performed during the acute TEN phase of conjunctival and corneal damages reduces the inflammatory process and prevents scarring [55, 63, 347, 348]. This procedure helps restoring corneal epithelial integrity and possibly prevent blindness [328, 329, 349-352].

19.2.1. Acute Stage

Suboptimal management of the ocular surface during the acute stage of TEN results in sight-threatening complication. Vigilant, intensive ocular management strategies in the acute TEN stage are essential. First, to switch off the acute ocular surface inflammatory response before it develops into persistent or chronic disease. Second, to protect the integrity of the ocular surface, facilitate healing, and minimize the risk of acute corneal perforation, and third to minimize and/or prevent symblepharon formation, progressive conjunctival scarring and chronic ocular surface failure.

Ocular hygiene is mandatory. Vigorous rinsing the eyes everyday with sterile saline removes any inflammatory debris from the ocular surface and lid margins, and helps decreasing the risk of ocular surface infection [321]. After the administration of topical anesthetic, local treatments include removal of pseudomembrane with a moist cotton tip, or a smooth blunt instrument, lysis of symblepharon using a glass rod and debridement of the loosened epithelium [62]. Controlling the destructive inflammation in the acute TEN phase probably prevents the long term ophthalmic events.

Early intensive topical corticosteroid drops or ointment may be safely used to help decreasing the acute TEN ocular surface damages. Betamethasone (0.1%) [55, 353] or dexamethasone (0.1%) [304] drops or fluorometholone ointment 0.1% [354] are generally used. The choice of a corticosteroid ointment (as opposed to solution) relies on the physical barrier provided by vehicle between denuded mucosal surfaces. Subconjunctival triamcinolone injections into the fornices (or subtarsus if the fornix is not accessible) are possibly used.

Topical cyclosporine (0.5%) possibly decreases the intensity of ocular surface inflammation in SJS and TEN, but no studies of this treatment currently exist [321, 353].

The ophthalmic management of acute SJS and TEN should focus on infections [355] prophylaxis using prophylactic topical antibiotics drops. Moxifloxacin 0.5% is bactericidal, effective against most common skin pathogens, and achieves high corneal and conjunctival concentrations [321]. Other typical infection prophylaxis regimen consist of bacitracin ointment and fluoroquinolone antibiotic. Immunosuppressive and antibiotics drops are generally applied sequentially at 2-hour intervals, 2 to 3 times a day. Combination tobramycin/dexamethasone ointment is generally applied to the eyelid margins and eyelashes at night.

Transplantation of cryopreserved AM suppresses inflammation, prevents ulcer formation and promotes healing during the acute stage of SJS and TEN, thus preventing sight-threatening cicatricial complications. Anatomically, AM is the innermost layer of the fetal membranes of the placenta. It consists of a single layer of epithelial cells bound to a thick basement membrane and a avascular stroma.

The rationale for use of AM in SJS and TEN is multifaceted. SJS and TEN involve variable degrees of sloughing of the conjunctival and corneal epithelial surfaces and attendant inflammation of the ocular surface. Coverage of these surfaces with AM creates a physical barrier between inflamed, denuded mucosal surfaces. Second, AM application confers an anti-inflammatory effect. Furthermore, AM exhibits potent antifibrotic effects. It also promotes limbal epithelial stem cell expansion [56, 351].

AM suppress innate immunity by trapping both macrophages and neutrophils within its stromal matrix and inducing them to undergo rapid apoptosis. AM downregulates T-helper cytokines secreted by activated lymphocytes and several pro-inflammatory cytokines, such as TNF and IL-6 secreted by activated macrophages. In addition, AM stromal matrix exerts a powerful direct anti-scarring action on ocular surface fibroblasts by suppressing TGF-β signalling at the transcriptional level, leading to downregulation of several downstream genes that are responsible for scar formation. Intriguingly, these therapeutic actions can also be delivered by cryopreserved AM used as a temporary biologic bandage even if it is acellular and contains no stem cells. Finally, AM application appears to confer beneficial effects on re-epithelialization the process beyond that afforded by a bandage contact lens alone, possibly by providing a scaffold for the migration of epithelial cells.

Whenever possible, AM should be applied under operating microscope and general anesthesia in an operating room. Intravenous sedation and analgesia should be used to augment anesthesia applied to the eyelids and ocular surface.

Although the most secure adhesion of AM to the ocular surface is obtained by use of sutures, alternative application techniques [351] have been described using biologic adhesive.

Not all SJS and TEN patients with ocular involvement develop serious sequelae. Patients with signs of intense or worsening inflammation of the conjunctiva and lid margins should be considered for treatment with AM transplantation. In this regard, lesions to be considered, are membranous conjunctivitis, early symblepharon formation, and intense lid margin inflammation with lash loss. Any of these suggest that severity in destructive inflammation puts the patient at a high risk for ocular surface scarring and severe dry eye problems. These patients report prominent ocular discomfort and photophobia. Extensive corneal epithelial defects are of concern, but they are partly related to exposure keratopathy, if the patient is sedated and on a ventilator.

Patients with moderate, nonmembranous conjunctivitis and minimal lid margin involvement need close daily monitoring with careful inspection of the fornices and tarsal conjunctiva for hidden inflammation of symblepharon. The described medical treatments should be implemented. Localized conjunctival epithelial defects are common in these patients and should be measured each day with use of fluorescein staining. Most digital cameras allow detailed bedside photographs of the defects to help documenting any changes. Handheld direct ophthalmoscopes are helpful for highlighting the fluorescein stain and for illuminating the eye for photos. Any signs of progressively worsening inflammation or expanding epithelial defects should warrant consideration for treatment with AM.

The membranes degrade over 10-14 days with lid margin and corneal portions breaking down first. As the membrane degrade, they commonly evoke mucopurulent discharge and araise concern about superinfection. At 10-14 days after the placement of the AM, the sutures are removed. Any areas that remain significantly inflamed are retreated. Special priority is given to the lid margins and tarsal conjunctiva, as scarring of these structures is particularly associated with long-term ocular morbidity. Some patients require up to three separate applications of AM over the course of a month due to persistent severe conjunctival inflammation.

19.2.2. Chronic Stage

Many patients with acute SJS and TEN fail to receive needed interventions during the acute phase. This occurs for a variety of reasons, including delayed ophthalmic care, lack of a standard evaluation and treatment protocol, and access to materials (i.e. AM). Therefore, opththalmologists often face the challenging task of treating patients with chronic, potentially blinding cicatricial ocular surface changes such as corneal epithelial defects and ulceration, corneal scarring, conjunctival scarring, symblepharon and limbal stem cell deficiency. Treatments for chronic sequelae have improved over the years, but most therapies continue to have limited success rates, both visually and symptomatically.

These treatments include a variety of topical medications, special contact lenses, conjunctival replacement procedures, limbal stem cell transplantation and keratoprostheses.

A "triple-TEN" management procedure was offered for the management of ocular complications of TEN in order to minimize the risk of blinding sequelae [356]. The triple-TEN protocol comprises (a) subconjunctival triamcinolone administered into each of the fornices to curb the local inflammatory response without compromising systemic immunity, (b) placement of amniotic membrane tissue mounted on a polycarbonate skirt over the corneal and limbal regions to facilitate reepithelialization of the ocular surface, and (c) insertion of a steeply curved acrylic scleral shell spacer to vault the lids away from the globe providing a barrier to symblepharon formation.

Chapter 20

Systemic Pharmacotherapy

For years, the trial-and-error approach to medical innovation for treating TEN was the only way of progress in the clinical practice. A new era has emerged when physicians and researchers got some tools for investigating the biologic reasons behind the therapeutic successes or failures.

In recent years, new TEN treatments have been attempted, but they often remained disappointing [43, 357-359]. A note of caution remains to be addressed in that field of diseases. In severe ADR, some potent treatments are occasionally more deleterious than beneficial, and they possibly add new injuries. The clinical diagnosis of sepsis is tough, and the decision to administer systemic antibiotics has to be carefully considered.

Several treatments appear beneficial in small sets of case reports and uncontrolled series. However, no undisputable evaluations exist, and clear indications from the literature are lacking for establishing any optimal individual treatment regimen. Currently, multi-agent therapies are probably indicated, targeting a set of likely intermediary mechanisms. These measures include residual offending drug removal, immunosuppression, inhibition of DR pathways, general antiapoptotic strategies, and aggressive supportive care. Particular attention is directed at avoiding potential conflicts between different treatments, and discarding any agent that theoretically exerts a net proapoptotic rather than antiapoptotic effect.

There is some evidence that one of the initial processes in TEN is immunological. Hence, there is good reason to consider using immunosuppressive agents in TEN treatment. However, a general concern about the use of immunosuppressors is the risk of promoting sepsis.

For severe ocular lesions, systemic immunosuppression with corticosteroids [354] and/or steroid sparing agents (cyclosporine, azathioprine, mycophenalate, cyclosphorphamide, adalimumab, infliximab, dapsone) are potentially considered in both SJS and TEN. Treatment guidelines are similar to those used in autoimmune bullous disorders. Topical corticosteroids are useful for controlling bouts of inflammation in chronic ocular surface disease, but their long-term use carries concern for cataract formation and glaucoma.

20.1. Glucocorticosteroids

A series of therapeutic modalities target various toxic mediators in TEN. They are beneficial for the management of patients. A notable example is provided by systemic corticosteroids. They represent immunosuppressive agents that were administered as a mainstay of the SJS and TEN treatment for several decades [103, 360]. Such treatment was supported by the pro-inflammatory effects of the toxic mediators involved in the TEN pathogenesis. Its use has been much debated and remains controversial.

Corticosteroids are highly potent agents targeting several intracellular processes and abating most facets of the inflammatory and immune response. Effects pertinent to TEN are on immunosuppression and control of apoptosis. Glucocorticoids inhibit T-cell activation via inhibition of IL-2 transcription through inhibition of transcription factor AP-1. A further key inhibited transcription factor is NF-κB involved in the regulation of production of many immunoregulatory and proinflammatory cytokines including IL-16, IL-8, IL-11, IL-12, IL-15, IL-16 and, of particular relevance, IFN-γ and TNF.

Whereas corticosteroids are proapoptotic in lymphoid cells, many hematopoietic cells and chondrocytes, they have been reported to be antiapoptotic in most other tissues including skin. One mechanism of this effect is inhibition of initiating pathways such as downregulation of FasR/FasL in the apoptotic tissue. In a model system of cocultured activated T cells and keratinocytes, apoptosis in keratinocytes was induced by lymphocytes secreting IFN-γ and sFasL. This process was inhibited by high dose of dexamethasone [361, 362], as well as cyclosporine, rapamycin and tacrolimus.

Corticosteroids potentially exhibit beneficial anti-inflammatory, immuno-suppressive and antiapoptotic effects. However, a drawback is the ability to downregulate NF-kB activity, particularly in the presence of abundant TNF. As with other causes of downregulation of NF-κB, downregulation by corticosteroids might result in apoptosis in the presence of TNF, although the combination of TNF and dexamethasone inhibits IFN-γ/anti-Fas antibody-mediated apoptosis in lung epithelial cells. However, there remain concerns that in TEN, the inhibition of NF-κB by corticosteroids probably results in a proapoptotic effect.

The proponents of corticotherapy in TEN patients consider that the early administration of systemic corticosteroids reduces the mortality rate without increasing time to healing.

Other authors reported no differences in mortality rates and infectious complications in corticosteorid treated TEN patients compared to those out of these drugs before admission in a burn unit. However, TEN is occasionally reported in patients under long-term corticotherapy before TEN onset. It is possible that corticosteroids delay the TEN onset, but fails to block its progression. Some studies showed that systemic corticotherapy for more than 48 h was detrimental associated with a five-fold increase in incidence of infection (especially *Candida* sepsis), a two-fold increase in the duration of hospitalization, and a 12.5-fold increase in mortality rate, independently of age, as well as in extent in epidermal sloughing, and in leukocyte count nadir.

According to these contrasting features, corticosteroids could be administered as a TEN treatment at the erythroderma stage before obvious skin loss occurrence.

In such restricted conditions, high doses of oral or parenteral dexamethasone [361, 362], prednisone or prednisolone could possibly be administered on admission as a pulse therapy [363]. However, such treatment should not be administered for more than 48 h since a prolonged period of corticotherapy is associated with a dramatic increase in TEN morbidity and mortality. Moreover, when over 20% of TBSA has sloughed, steroid therapy is contraindicated due to increased risk of sepsis. The major limitation of corticotherapy is due to the fact that it often remains difficult to diagnose TEN at the initial non-bullous stage.

The balance of the current evidence suggests that, at best, corticosteroids have no major beneficial effect in TEN patients, and, at worst, are detrimental. Coupled with the theoretical concerns outlined above, corticosteroids are not recommended as an outstanding therapy for TEN patients.

20.2. Intravenous Immunoglobulins

The rationale for pooled human IVIg administrations to TEN patients relies on the presence of IgG antibodies directed to CD95R in commercial IVIg batches [364]. They are expected to settle in part inside the epidermis [365, 366] blocking the FasL binding to FasR. Such mechanism is in line with the concept considering that keratinocyte FasL ligation of FasR is the mechanism for apoptosis in TEN. An alternative interpretation of FasL expression by keratinocytes suggests a defence mechanism against immune attack involving ligation of FasR on lymphocytes. This concept implies apoptosis of lymphoid cells rather than keratinocytes. An alternative hypothesis considers that the source of FasL is blood mononuclear cells rather than keratinocytes [223]. Few FasL is detected on keratinocytes in TEN, but high serum levels of sFasL, are increased when blood mononuclear cells are exposed to the causative drug. Sera of patients with TEN and SJS induce abundant keratinocyte apoptosis.

Treatment of TEN with IVIg has been reported in several case series, with conflicting results. Several series supported the use of IVIg, reporting reduced mortality rates from the disease [364-367]. Other data were less encouraging. These studies were difficult to compare because of the wide variation in patients and treatment protocols. Various commercial brands of IVIg have been used, and different dosing regimens applied. IVIg are a diverse product developed from the pooled serum of hundreds of blood donors. Wide batch-to-batch variation in anti-Fas activity in vitro has been demonstrated, and not all the contents and their biological activities are known. Although data suggest that IVIg may be of use in TEN, study results are conflicting [368-377].

A series of prospective and retrospective studies, as well as meta-analysis, have assessed the limited benefit of IVIg in TEN treatment. Conflicting outcomes were reported in several case series, suggesting either reduction in the mortality rate or, conversely, no beneficial effect in comparison with supportive care only [358]. IVIg do not appear to reduce the severity of ocular complications. Differences in anti-CD95R activity in IVIg batches, at usual IVIg doses (doses over 2 g/kg are expected to reduce mortality), and/or time from TEN onset to the IVIg administration possibly contribute to the different outcomes. A beneficial effect were observed in the TEN damages in the eyes of some patients [378].

There is no strong evidence supporting IVIg administration in TEN. Subgroups of patients, if any, who could benefit from this treatment should be identified. Indeed, IVIg do not curb the mortality rate when the SCORTEN risk of mortality is high.

20.3. Cyclosporine A

Cyclosporine A (CSA) is a potent immunomodulator that was advocated as a potential agent for reversing TEN progression [379-382]. The suppressive action of CSA is blockade of T cell activation and proliferation by selective inhibition of calcineurin. The CSA immunosuppressive effects inhibitory effect on CD8+ CTC is associated with the partial inhibition of the activation of macrophages and CD95 system. In vitro, CSA abates the drug-induced expression of FasR and FasL mRNA, and blocks drug-mediated apoptosis in some cell types [383]. However, CSA does not inhibit the cytolytic capacity of activated CD8+ CTC.

Only a few and uncontrolled TEN cases have been treated with CSA. Beneficial effects were generally reported. The effects of CSA (5 mg/kg/day) on the epidermis of TEN patients were compared to those obtained with supportive care only. Similarly to the IVIg findings, the apoptosis marker CD95R was downregulated in clinically involved TEN skin at completion of a 5-day CSA treatment [384]. This finding clinically confirmed the in vitro inhibitory effect of CSA on the CD95 system. No significant effect of CSA was evidenced on the extent of the TEN inflammatory cell infiltrate. This might be surprising because CSA exerts a potent inhibitory effect on activated T lymphocytes. However, the inability of CSA to reduce the skin accumulation of an inflammatory cell infiltrate was previously noticed in alopecia areata [385]. In comparison with supportive care alone CSA treatment did not improve the reepithelialization and did not significantly decrease morbidity and mortality in TEN. It is also noteworthy that TEN occasionally develop in patients having previously received CSA for other clinical disorders.

In sum, CSA treatment has a number of potential benefits in TEN. It is strongly immunosuppressive and antiapoptotic, and does not downreglate NF-κB, although there may be some inhibition of TNF. It partly inhibits the CD95 system in TEN patients. However, this drug does not appear powerful enough in some patients to initiate a clinically relevant improvement in TEN prognosis.

20.4. Anti-TNF Antibodies

The putative pathogenic importance of TNF in TEN suggests an innovative therapeutic approach consisting of a selective blockade of using specific antibodies. So far, only a few case reports described the successful treatment of TEN patients with anti-TNF antibodies. Only a few patients were treated with infliximab [386-389] (at a dose of 3 or 5 mg/kg in a one-shot intravenous perfusion of 2 h) or etanercept (one subcutaneous injection of 25 mg administrated 4 and 8 days post-admission) [390]. In each patient, the treatment stopped the rapid progression of the disease. There were no specific adverse effects increased susceptibility to infection. Immunohistochemistry showed that 24 h after anti-TNF therapy, immunoreactivity for TNF was markedly decreased in lesional skin [296]. In correlation with protein immunoreactivity, TNF mRNA expression dramatically decreased after anti-TNF therapy. The efficacy of this treatment is to be confirmed in larger groups of TEN patients.

The anti-TNF and anti IL-6 thalidomide was reported to have a deleterious effect in the condition [391], which would be compatible with active TNF antiapoptotic pathways. This raises questions about the suitability of any treatment for TEN that might downregulate the TNF-NF-kB pathway.

20.5. N-acetylcysteine

N-acetylcysteine (NAC) is a cysteine derivative precursor of GSH [392]. A NAC treatment is possibly effective in severe drug reactions according to three mechanisms: a) reacting with oxidative compounds and replenishing intracellular cysteine levels for the production of GSH, b) blocking the expression of the homing receptor for CLA, and c) inhibiting the production of TNF and IL-1 [393, 394]. In addition, NAC increases the clearance of several drugs and their metabolites. A few patients were successfully treated with high-dose intravenous NAC in open studies [392]. However, a randomized trial did not confirm the efficacy of NAC in the prevention of hypersensitivity reactions to trimethoprim-sulfamethoxazole in patients with HIV infection. Moreover, high doses of NAC may inactivate not only the culprit drug but also other drugs potentially useful for the patients [393]. The combination of NAC and TNF-a inhibitor failed to improve the patient survival [394].

20.6. Other Immunomodulators

Pentoxifylline [395], cyclosphosphamide [396], granulocyte macrophage colony-stimulating factor (GMCSF) [397], thalidomide and ulinastatin (urinary trypsin inhibitor) [398] were used in a few case reports. The lack of controlled studies and their putative mode of action make it difficult to propose them as appropriate treatments for TEN.

20.7. Plasmapheresis and Hemodialysis

Plasmapheresis and hemodialysis aim at enhanced removal the offending drug, its metabolites or other toxic mediators including harmful cytokines from the blood circulation. They have been used to alleviate the manifestations of SJS and TEN [399-401]. Small molecules, including most drugs, are readily filtered, provided they are not heavily bound to proteins like albumin. Plasmapheresis would be expected to be more effective in respect of cytokine clearance. Molecules up to 40 kDa are filtered. The TNF monomer is 17 kDa, but TNF typically exists as a trimer with a molecular weight of 54 kDa. FasL is structurally similar and forms a trimer.

Plasmapheresis was used singly or in association with IVIg, with some beneficial and promising results in TEN [399-401]. Plasmapheresis is supposed to remove any drug accumulation, its metabolites and cytotoxic mediators. However, plasmapheresis does not always substantially decrease blood and tissue cytokines. Indeed, the natural production and degradation of cytokines are often too fast to be effectively controlled by this method [399]. Moreover, removal of plasma calls for substitution fluid containing a suitable amount of fresh frozen plasma. Such replacement is costly and, if sustained for long periods of time, represents a serious burden on the local blood bank. In addition, plasmapheresis removes soluble pro- and anti-inflammatory mediators simultaneously, which can negatively modify the patient's immunity [404]. It needs a vascular access which is a potential source of infection in TEN. Some authors believe that plasma exchanges do not show a significant therapeutic effect in TEN [397]. In sum, the lack of controlled studies, even regarding the mechanism of action of plasmapheresis makes it difficult to determine its true efficacy [405].

Chapter 21

Tissue Replacement

21.1. Conjunctival Replacement

In chronic SJS and TEN eyelid disease, the condition is often severe and represents a major causal factor in the progression of corneal decompensation through mechanical microtrauma [63]. Eyelid disease is often linked to advanced cicatricial changes of the conjunctiva. It includes cicatricial entropion/ectropion, trichiasis, lid margin keratinization, tarsal keratinization scarring and symblepharon.

Manual epilation, electrolysis, laser and cryoablative methods are used to address misdirection of the eyelashes. Lagophtalmos is conveniently treated by lysis of scar tissue or by tarsorrhaphy. Autologous oral mucosal grafts is possibly used to reshape the fornix in cases of severe symblepharon or to rebuilt the lid margins in cases of lid margin keratinization. However, the scarring response after surgery is occasionally quite severe, given the loss of normal mucosal architecture, and recurrence of adhesions is common.

21.2. Corneal Replacement

Facing a major limbal SCD, with extensive corneal neovascularization and/or persistent corneal epithelial defects, an autologous or allogeneic limbal stem cell transplant is encouraged to stabilize the ocular surface. Because limbal stem cell deficiency is usually bilateral in SJS and TEN, visual rehabilitation efforts are limited to transplantation of allogeneic limbal stem cells. Due to continuous ocular surface changes and other cicatricial complications, eyes with total limbal SCD caused by SJS and TEN convey the worst prognosis, even after transplantation of allogeneic limbal stem cells.

When allogeneic tissue is transferred, the patients require prolonged, potentially indefinite systemic immunosuppression typically including tacrolimus and mycophenolate mofetil. Promising results were reported following transplantation of cultivated oral mucosa epithelial in case of total limbal SCD.

In obvious corneal opacification, a corneal transplant is considered after an attempt at limbal stem cell transplantation. Moreover, in the presence of severe dry eye, inflammation, and eyelid scarring, such surgical process is at high risk for failure. When a corneal transplant fails or in case of advanced corneal scarring, an artificial cornea, such as a type I or II Boston keratoprosthesis [406], or an osteo-odonto-keratoprosthesis should be considered associated or not with a limbal stem cell transplant. The type I Boston device is a collar button device of polymethylmethacrylate and titanium inserted through the centre of a donor cornea, and sutured onto the eye in a procedure similar to a traditional penetrating keratoplasty. The type II device is placed through the permanently closed upper eyelid and cornea in a more extensive procedure. Keratoprothesis in SJS and TEN commonly have better outcome than with penetrating keratoplasty, but it is not as good as its use in nonautoimmune cases. Melting around the devices, extrusion glaucoma and endophthalmitis are not uncommon. However, although patients with autoimmune diseases carry the worst prognosis, keratoprothesis implantation potentially evolves into a viable option for those patients exhibiting the most serious long-term sequelae in ocular SJS and TEN.

Chapter 22

Cost-Effectiveness of Treatment

The development of a disease management approach to the care of severe ADR is driven by medical and economic considerations. Currently, state-of-the-art ADR therapy involves several treatment modalities that are provided by different medical professionals with the hope of providing better wound healing status for patients. When the integration of these decision-making planning and care provision modalitites is less than optimal, one has to expect poor health outcomes.

The cost-effectiveness of the TEN treatment is not a matter of importance. The disease is so rare that there is no impact on the general health cost. The matter of concern is purely medical with the hope of increasing the survival of patients. The situation is similar to that encountered in extensive PTTB patients. From an economic point of view, care providers cannot supply indistinctly in different populations whatever interventions are theoretically possible but not actually available at a given regional scale. Rising health care costs in absence of an efficient health security system, probably determines the level and extent of care that can be provided to patients. The system has a say in every aspect of therapy, from where it should be provided by whom to which technologies should be used.

Scleral lenses and surgical procedures on the damaged eyes are expensive, but are usually rewarding in the repair process of severe ocular lesions. It remains that current treatments commonly provide partial and temporary relief. They are prone to failures.

Part IV: Framing the Future

Chapter 23

Spotlight on Perspective

This monograph is a digest of the knowledge of nearly all current authorities on TEN. A pitfall in skin research is the danger of losing sight of the whole in a sincere, if somewhat misguided, search for the parts. Indeed, a variety of pathomechanisms are involved in necrolytic blistering diseases. TEN is a typical example of such a wide diversity. Keratinocytes appear to be prominent mediators in the epidermal destruction in TEN. A combined process of apoptosis and necrosis is likely initiated by an altered detoxication pathway of the offending drug inside these cells. TEN pathomechanisms lead to an enzymatic chain reaction with the production of different interactive proinflammatory cytokines in the epidermis. So far, no single specific treatment has proven to be highly active in TEN. None of them appears significantly superior to supportive care only. It is suggested that several molecular targets blocking different apoptosis/necrosis pathways should be hit simultaneously in the keratinocytes in order to reach real efficacy in TEN treatment.

The disruption of the mitochondrial electron transfer chain by electrophilic metabolites of the offending drug could represent a major step leading to both early apoptosis and late necrosis in TEN. Accordingly, the recovery of the electron transport chain possibly represents a key target in TEN control. Treatments only blocking the effects of the proinflammatory cytokines and receptors produced in TEN, without acting on the deregulation of the mitochondrial electron transport chain likely exert a limited effect on the TEN course. This is the case for the current monotherapies using compounds such as IVIg, systemic corticosteroids, cyclosporine and anti-TNF agents. As the pace of biotechnological innovation accelerates major progresses are expected in a near future.

Any attempt to establish evidence-based medicine recommendations is hampered by the rare occurrence of TEN in the population. The TEN treatments which received the more attention from clinicians are high-dose systemic glucocorticoids and IVIg. The former treatment is associated with potentially disastrous adverse effects. The latter treatment has proven biological effects, but does not seem to be able to fully reverse TEN evolution. However, IVIg might be useful in some TEN patients and are not generally prone to adverse effects. Based on the putative TEN pathomechanism, the use of anti-TNF antibodies is a promising approach to TEN treatment, but new antiapoptotic molecules acting on keratinocytes are undoubtedly needed. Until effective chemical treatments are developed to neutralize the reactive electrophilic metabolites, and to restore the electron transfer chain in TEN keratinocytes, several blocking agents (e.g. NAC combined with IVIg or TNF antagonists) failed to improve the issue of TEN.

In spite of being uncommon, SJS and TEN have a major impact on public health by virtue of high mortality. Unfortunately, there is no treatment guideline highlighting the inadequacy of current treatment regimens. The rationale for recent therapeutic interventions of SJS/TEN is mainly derived from empiric evidence regarding the understanding of cytotoxic pathways in keratinocytes and lymphocytes elicited by drug exposure. It is conceivable that a novel treatment for combating granulysin-mediated cell death alone or in combination with existing agents will be beneficial to achieve a better outcome in unfortunate people who suffer from this deadly adverse drug reaction.

Caution is necessary in initiating such trials, since previous studies have demonstrated that some theorically useful molecules in TEN, such a thalidomide, have increased the mortality in clinical conditions. Some readers are probably surprised at how little firm data is available to aid in making recommendations for TEN management. Moreover, the relevance of new clinical trials will probably be questioned in TEN owing to the rarity and the severity of the disease. Such situation hardly permits to organize safe double-blind studies with adequate statistical power.

It is clear that controversies are present in the interpretations of clinical findings. Many fruitful areas of research remain open. Forthcoming information from different fields with varying approaches will certainly lead to cross-fertilization of ideas and mutual advances.

TEN is a rare but serious dermatological disorder with significant mortality, highlighting the inadequacy of current accepted treatments. Much work still needs to be done to elucidate the pathogenesis of TEN fully and to establish more effective therapy. Recent developments in our understanding of apoptotic pathways in keratinocytes and lymphocytes, and of specific immunological changes related to drug reactions, offer intriguing insights.

One aspect of the future is offered by keratinocyte grafting of the wound areas to restore an essential barrier between the living tissues of the body and the external environment. Any large interruption in the skin is life-threatening. Allogeneic cells are inexorably immunologically rejected. Cultured epithelial autografts take at least 3 weeks to grow enough cells for successful grafting, due to the low number of keratinocyte stem cells recovered from skin biopsies. Alternative sources of cells for engineering skin substitutes are urgently required to address this area of clinical need. One possibility is to use fetal skin as a potential cell source for tissue-engineered skin. Indeed, fetal keratinocytes have faster expansion times, longer telomeres, and lower immunogenicity indicators.

Combining the current available evidence relating to the efficacy of treatments, and the likely pathogenic mechanisms, certain conclusions can be drawn. All patients should be admitted to a specialist high dependency/intensive care unit as soon as the diagnosis has been established, for full assessment and expert multidisciplinary supportive therapy. All possible offending or triggering drugs should be stopped. There is a strong case for immediate hemofiltration to remove any residual causative drug, and to reduce proapoptotic cytokine levels. TEN appears immunologically mediated and early use of a powerful immunosuppressive would seem indicated. A potential problem with immunosuppression is that secondary infection, which is a major complication of TEN, is potentially precipitated or exacerbated. However, TEN currently has a high mortality and it is essential to combat the pathogenic process. Based on the current knowledge and the theoretical discussion outlined above, cyclosporine would seem to be an immunosuppressor of choice. IVIg have been extensively used but their value has not been definitely determined. A specific anti-FasL antibody, if developed in the future, may be of greater value. Insulin is now routinely used in the critical care environment to maintain strict normoglycemia, and ill patients with TEN are likely to need it. There is a case for early recourse to this treatment in TEN in view of its antiapoptotic potential. Multicentre studies are needed to look further at potentially promising treatment combinations.

References

[1] Lyell, A. Toxic epidermal necrolysis: an eruption resembling scalding of the skin. *Br J Dermatol* 1956; 68: 355-361.

[2] Lyell, A. Requiem for toxic epidermal necrolysis. *Br J Dermatol* 1990; 122: 837-838.

[3] Forman, R; Koren, G; Shear, NH. Erythema multiforme, Stevens-Johnson syndrome and toxic epidermal necrolysis in children: a review of 10 years' experience. *Drug Saf* 2002; 25: 965-972.

[4] Prendiville, J. Stevens-Johnson syndrome and toxic epidermal necrolysis. *Adv Dermatol* 2002; 18: 151-173.

[5] Wolf, R; Wolf, D; Davidovici, B. In the pursuit of classifying severe cutaneous adverse reactions. *Clin Dermatol* 2007; 25: 348-349.

[6] Paquet, P; Piérard, GE. New insights in toxic epidermal necrolysis (Lyell's syndrome): clinical considerations, pathobiology and targeted treatments revisited. *Drug Saf* 2010; 33: 189-212.

[7] Ducic, I; Shalom, A; Rising, W, et al. Outcome of patients with toxic epidermal necrolysis syndrome revisited. *Plast Reconstr Surg* 2002; 110: 768-773.

[8] Schneck, J; Fagot, JP; Sekula, P, et al. Effects of treatments on the mortality of Stevens-Johnson syndrome and toxic epidermal necrolysis: A retrospective study on patients included in the prospective EuroSCAR Study. *J Am Acad Dermatol* 2008; 58: 33-40.

[9] Piérard, GE; Paquet, P. Facing up to toxic epidermal necrolysis. *Expert Opin Pharmacother* 2010; 11: 2443-2446.

[10] Gravante, G; Esposito, G; Delogu, D, et al. More than two different bacterial species isolated from blood of toxic epidermal necrolysis patients significantly increase mortality. *Burns* 2006; 32: 793-794.

[11] Jin, H; Qiao, J; Wang, B, et al. Toxic epidermal necrolysis complicated by Mucor infection. *Int J Dermatol* 2008; 47: 383-386.
[12] de Prost, N; Ingen-Housz-Oro, S; Duong, T, et al. Bacteremia in Stevens-Johnson syndrome and toxic epidermal necrolysis: epidemiology, risk factors, and predictive value of skin cultures. *Medicine (Baltimore)* 2010; 89: 28-36.
[13] Fritsch, PO; Sidoroff, A. Drug-induced Stevens-Johnson syndrome/toxic epidermal necrolysis. *Am J Clin Dermatol* 2000; 1: 349-360.
[14] Schulz, JT; Sheridan, RL; Ryan, CM, et al. A 10-year experience with toxic epidermal necrolysis. *J Burn Care Rehabil* 2000; 21: 199-204.
[15] Noël, JC; Buxant, F; Fayt, I, et al. Vulval adenosis associated with toxic epidermal necrolysis. *Br J Dermatol* 2005; 153: 457-458.
[16] Pereira, FA; Mudgil, AV; Rosmarin, DM. Toxic epidermal necrolysis. *J Am Acad Dermatol* 2007; 56: 181-200.
[17] Abood, GJ; Nickoloff, BJ; Gamelli, RL. Treatment strategies in toxic epidermal necrolysis syndrome: where are we at? *J Burn Care Res* 2008; 29: 269-276.
[18] Gerull, R; Nelle, M; Schaible, T. Toxic epidermal necrolysis and Stevens-Johnson syndrome: a review. *Crit Care Med* 2011; 39: 1521-1532.
[19] Castelain, F; Humbert, P. Toxic epidermal necrolysis. *Curr Drug Saf* 2012; 7: 332-338.
[20] Harr, T; French, LE. Stevens-Johnson syndrome and toxic epidermal necrolysis. *Chem Immunol Allergy* 2012; 97: 149-166.
[21] Saka, B; Barro-Traore, F; Atadokpede, FA, et al. Stevens-Johnson syndrome and toxic epidermal necrolysis in sub-Saharan Africa: a multicentric study in four countries. *Int J Dermatol* 2013; 52: 575-579.
[22] Schwartz, RA; McDonough, PH; Lee, BW. Toxic epidermal necrolysis: Part I. Introduction, history, classification, clinical features, systemic manifestations, etiology, and immunopathogenesis. *J Am Acad Dermatol* 2013; 69: 173 e171-113; quiz 185-176.
[23] Schwartz, RA; McDonough, PH; Lee, BW. Toxic epidermal necrolysis: Part II. Prognosis, sequelae, diagnosis, differential diagnosis, prevention, and treatment. *J Am Acad Dermatol* 2013; 69: 187 e181-116; quiz 203-184.
[24] Piérard-Franchimont, C; Quatresooz, P; Reginster, MA, et al. Finding the drug in cutaneous drug eruptions. *Rev Med Liege* 2011; 66: 474-477.
[25] Hermanns-Lê, T; Piérard-Franchimont, C; Piérard, GE. The spectrum of drug eruptions. *Rev Med Liege* 2013; 68: 44-50.

[26] Endorf, FW; Cancio, LC; Gibran, NS. Toxic epidermal necrolysis clinical guidelines. *J Burn Care Res* 2008; 29: 706-712.

[27] Mulvey, JM; Padowitz, A; Lindley-Jones, M, et al. Mycoplasma pneumoniae associated with Stevens Johnson syndrome. *Anaesth Intensive Care* 2007; 35: 414-417.

[28] Neuman, MG; McKinney, KK; Nanau, RM, et al. Drug-induced severe adverse reaction enhanced by human herpes virus-6 reactivation. *Transl Res* 2013; 161: 430-440.

[29] Downey, A; Jackson, C; Harun, N, et al. Toxic epidermal necrolysis: review of pathogenesis and management. *J Am Acad Dermatol* 2012; 66: 995-1003.

[30] Webb, DV; Stowman, AM; Patterson, JW. Boric acid ingestion clinically mimicking toxic epidermal necrolysis. *J Cutan Pathol* 2013; 40: 962-965.

[31] Reilly, TP; Lash, LH; Doll, MA, et al. A role for bioactivation and covalent binding within epidermal keratinocytes in sulfonamide-induced cutaneous drug reactions. *J Invest Dermatol* 2000; 114: 1164-1173.

[32] Baron, JM; Merk, HF. Drug metabolism in the skin. *Curr Opin Allergy Clin Immunol* 2001; 1: 287-291.

[33] Vyas, PM; Roychowdhury, S; Koukouritaki, SB, et al. Enzyme-mediated protein haptenation of dapsone and sulfamethoxazole in human keratinocytes: II. Expression and role of flavin-containing monooxygenases and peroxidases. *J Pharmacol Exp Ther* 2006; 319: 497-505.

[34] Dietrich, A; Kawakubo, Y; Rzany, B, et al. Low N-acetylating capacity in patients with Stevens-Johnson syndrome and toxic epidermal necrolysis. *Exp Dermatol* 1995; 4: 313-316.

[35] Paquet, P; Jacob, E; Pirson, J, et al. Drug-induced toxic epidermal necrolysis and pancytopenia: a puzzling association. *Int J Mol Med* 2005; 16: 29-33.

[36] Paquet, P; Nikkels, A; Arrese, JE, et al. Macrophages and tumor necrosis factor alpha in toxic epidermal necrolysis. *Arch Dermatol* 1994; 130: 605-608.

[37] Paquet, P; Piérard, GE. Keratinocyte injury in drug-induced toxic epidermal necrolysis: Simultaneous but distinct topographic expression of CD95R and calprotectin. *Int J Mol Med* 2002; 10: 145-147.

[38] Franchimont, C; Piérard, GE. Cutaneous pathobiology mediated by chemotherapy. *J Cutan Pathol* 1980; 7: 387-393.

[39] Piérard-Franchimont, C; Lesuisse, M; Humbert, P, et al. Toxic epidermal necrolysis and antifolate drugs in cancer chemotherapy. *Curr Drug Saf* 2012; 7: 357-360.

[40] Halevi, A; Ben-Amitai, D; Garty, BZ. Toxic epidermal necrolysis associated with acetaminophen ingestion. *Ann Pharmacother* 2000; 34: 32-34.

[41] Chave, TA; Mortimer, NJ; Sladden, MJ, et al. Toxic epidermal necrolysis: current evidence, practical management and future directions. *Br J Dermatol* 2005; 153: 241-253.

[42] Tohyama, M; Hashimoto, K. Immunological mechanisms of epidermal damage in toxic epidermal necrolysis. *Curr Opin Allergy Clin Immunol* 2012; 12: 376-382.

[43] Khalili, B; Bahna, SL. Pathogenesis and recent therapeutic trends in Stevens-Johnson syndrome and toxic epidermal necrolysis. *Ann Allergy Asthma Immunol* 2006; 97: 272-280; quiz 281-273, 320.

[44] Posadas, SJ; Padial, A; Torres, MJ, et al. Delayed reactions to drugs show levels of perforin, granzyme B, and Fas-L to be related to disease severity. *J Allergy Clin Immunol* 2002; 109: 155-161.

[45] Posadas, SJ; Torres, MJ; Mayorga, C, et al. Gene expression levels of cytokine profile and cytotoxic markers in non-immediate reactions to drugs. *Blood Cells Mol Dis* 2002; 29: 179-189.

[46] Paquet, P; Piérard, GE. Erythema multiforme and toxic epidermal necrolysis: a comparative study. *Am J Dermatopathol* 1997; 19: 127-132.

[47] Redondo, P; Vicente, J; Espana, A, et al. Photo-induced toxic epidermal necrolysis caused by clobazam. *Br J Dermatol* 1996; 135: 999-1002.

[48] Paquet, P; Piérard, GE. Soluble fractions of tumor necrosis factor-alpha, interleukin-6 and of their receptors in toxic epidermal necrolysis: a comparison with second-degree burns. *Int J Mol Med* 1998; 1: 459-462.

[49] Correia, O; Delgado, L; Roujeau, JC, et al. Soluble interleukin 2 receptor and interleukin 1alpha in toxic epidermal necrolysis: a comparative analysis of serum and blister fluid samples. *Arch Dermatol* 2002; 138: 29-32.

[50] Paquet, P; Jacob, E; Piérard, GE. Cystic lesion of the parotid following drug-induced toxic epidermal necrolysis (Lyell's syndrome). *J Oral Pathol Med* 2005; 34: 380-382.

[51] Sibaud, V; Fricain, JC; Leaute-Labreze, C, et al. Persistant mucosal ulcerations: a rare complication of toxic epidermal necrolysis. *Ann Dermatol Venereol* 2005; 132: 682-685.

[52] Sedghizadeh, PP; Kumar, SK; Gorur, A, et al. Toxic epidermal necrolysis with a rare long-term oral complication requiring surgical intervention. *Oral Surg Oral Med Oral Pathol Oral Radiol Endod* 2008; 105: e29-33.

[53] Chang, YS; Huang, FC; Tseng, SH, et al. Erythema multiforme, Stevens-Johnson syndrome, and toxic epidermal necrolysis: acute ocular manifestations, causes, and management. *Cornea* 2007; 26: 123-129.

[54] Yip, LW; Thong, BY; Lim, J, et al. Ocular manifestations and complications of Stevens-Johnson syndrome and toxic epidermal necrolysis: an Asian series. *Allergy* 2007; 62: 527-531.

[55] Sotozono, C; Ueta, M; Koizumi, N, et al. Diagnosis and treatment of Stevens-Johnson syndrome and toxic epidermal necrolysis with ocular complications. *Ophthalmology* 2009; 116: 685-690.

[56] Hsu, M; Jayaram, A; Verner, R, et al. Indications and outcomes of amniotic membrane transplantation in the management of acute Stevens-Johnson syndrome and toxic epidermal necrolysis: a case-control study. *Cornea* 2012; 31: 1394-1402.

[57] Di Pascuale, MA; Espana, EM; Liu, DT, et al. Correlation of corneal complications with eyelid cicatricial pathologies in patients with Stevens-Johnson syndrome and toxic epidermal necrolysis syndrome. *Ophthalmology* 2005; 112: 904-912.

[58] De Rojas, MV; Dart, JK; Saw, VP. The natural history of Stevens Johnson syndrome: patterns of chronic ocular disease and the role of systemic immunosuppressive therapy. *Br J Ophthalmol* 2007; 91: 1048-1053.

[59] Schulze Schwering, M; Kayange, P; van Oosterhout, JJ, et al. Severe eye complications from Stevens-Johnson syndrome in a human immunodeficiency virus-infected patient in Malawi. *Am J Trop Med Hyg* 2013; 89: 162-164.

[60] Lopez-Garcia, JS; Rivas Jara, L; Garcia-Lozano, CI, et al. Ocular features and histopathologic changes during follow-up of toxic epidermal necrolysis. *Ophthalmology* 2011; 118: 265-271.

[61] Morales, ME; Purdue, GF; Verity, SM, et al. Ophthalmic Manifestations of Stevens-Johnson Syndrome and Toxic Epidermal Necrolysis and Relation to SCORTEN. *Am J Ophthalmol* 2010; 150: 505-510 e501.

[62] Fu, Y; Gregory, DG; Sippel, KC, et al. The ophthalmologist's role in the management of acute Stevens-Johnson syndrome and toxic epidermal necrolysis. *Ocul Surf* 2010; 8: 193-203.

[63] Lin, A; Patel, N; Yoo, D, et al. Management of ocular conditions in the burn unit: thermal and chemical burns and Stevens-Johnson syndrome/toxic epidermal necrolysis. *J Burn Care Res* 2011; 32: 547-560.

[64] Gueudry, J; Roujeau, JC; Binaghi, M, et al. Risk factors for the development of ocular complications of Stevens-Johnson syndrome and toxic epidermal necrolysis. *Arch Dermatol* 2009; 145: 157-162.

[65] Lebargy, F; Wolkenstein, P; Gisselbrecht, M, et al. Pulmonary complications in toxic epidermal necrolysis: a prospective clinical study. *Intensive Care Med* 1997; 23: 1237-1244.

[66] Hague, JS; Goulding, JM; Long, TM, et al. Respiratory involvement in toxic epidermal necrolysis portends a poor prognosis that may not be reflected in SCORTEN. *Br J Dermatol* 2007; 157: 1294-1296.

[67] de Prost, N; Mekontso-Dessap, A; Valeyrie-Allanore, L, et al. Acute respiratory failure in patients with toxic epidermal necrolysis: clinical features and factors associated with mechanical ventilation. *Crit Care Med* 2014; 42: 118-128.

[68] Barrera, JE; Meyers, AD; Hartford, EC. Hypopharyngeal stenosis and dysphagia complicating toxic epidermal necrolysis. *Arch Otolaryngol Head Neck Surg* 1998; 124: 1375-1376.

[69] Clayton, NA; Kennedy, PJ. Management of dysphagia in toxic epidermal necrolysis (TEN) and Stevens-Johnson syndrome (SJS). *Dysphagia* 2007; 22: 187-192.

[70] Kedward, AL; McKenna, K. A fatal case of toxic epidermal necrolysis with extensive intestinal involvement. *Clin Exp Dermatol* 2009; 34: e484.

[71] Sugimoto, Y; Mizutani, H; Sato, T, et al. Toxic epidermal necrolysis with severe gastrointestinal mucosal cell death: a patient who excreted long tubes of dead intestinal epithelium. *J Dermatol* 1998; 25: 533-538.

[72] Sakai, N; Yoshizawa, Y; Amano, A, et al. Toxic epidermal necrolysis complicated by multiple intestinal ulcers. *Int J Dermatol* 2008; 47: 180-182.

[73] Dylewski, ML; Prelack, K; Keaney, T, et al. Asymptomatic hyperamylasemia and hyperlipasemia in pediatric patients with toxic epidermal necrolysis. *J Burn Care Res* 2010; 31: 292-296.

[74] Blum, L; Chosidow, O; Rostoker, G, et al. Renal involvement in toxic epidermal necrolysis. *J Am Acad Dermatol* 1996; 34: 1088-1090.

[75] Hung, CC; Liu, WC; Kuo, MC, et al. Acute renal failure and its risk factors in Stevens-Johnson syndrome and toxic epidermal necrolysis. *Am J Nephrol* 2009; 29: 633-638.

[76] Meneux, E; Wolkenstein, P; Haddad, B, et al. Vulvovaginal involvement in toxic epidermal necrolysis: a retrospective study of 40 cases. *Obstet Gynecol* 1998; 91: 283-287.

[77] Niemeijer, IC; van Praag, MC; van Gemund, N. Relevance and consequences of erythema multiforme, Stevens-Johnson syndrome and toxic epidermal necrolysis in gynecology. *Arch Gynecol Obstet* 2009; 280: 851-854.

[78] Pacheco, H; Araujo, T; Kerdel, F. Toxic epidermal necrolysis in a pregnant, HIV-infected woman. *Int J Dermatol* 2002; 41: 600-601.

[79] Rodriguez, G; Trent, JT; Mirzabeigi, M, et al. Toxic epidermal necrolysis in a mother and fetus. *J Am Acad Dermatol* 2006; 55: S96-98.

[80] Struck, MF; Illert, T; Liss, Y, et al. Toxic epidermal necrolysis in pregnancy: case report and review of the literature. *J Burn Care Res* 2010; 31: 816-821.

[81] Huang, LY; Lin, CM; Chiou, CC, et al. Rhabdomyolysis as a potential complication of carbamazepine-induced toxic epidermal necrolysis. *Clin Biochem* 2012; 45: 1531-1532.

[82] Goens, J; Song, M; Fondu, P, et al. Haematological disturbances and immune mechanisms in toxic epidermal necrolysis. *Br J Dermatol* 1986; 114: 255-259.

[83] Samanci, N; Balci, N; Alpsoy, E. Heterotopic ossification related to toxic epidermal necrolysis in a patient with Behcet's disease. *J Dermatol* 2005; 32: 469-473.

[84] Kamada, N; Kinoshita, K; Togawa, Y, et al. Chronic pulmonary complications associated with toxic epidermal necrolysis: report of a severe case with anti-Ro/SS-A and a review of the published work. *J Dermatol* 2006; 33: 616-622.

[85] Sheridan, RL; Schulz, JT; Ryan, CM, et al. Long-term consequences of toxic epidermal necrolysis in children. *Pediatrics* 2002; 109: 74-78.

[86] Magina, S; Lisboa, C; Leal, V, et al. Dermatological and ophthalmological sequels in toxic epidermal necrolysis. *Dermatology* 2003; 207: 33-36.

[87] Paquet, P; Piérard, GE. Intense pulsed light treatment of persistent facial hypermelanosis following drug-induced toxic epidermal necrolysis. *Dermatol Surg* 2004; 30: 1522-1525.

[88] Haber, J; Hopman, W; Gomez, M, et al. Late outcomes in adult survivors of toxic epidermal necrolysis after treatment in a burn center. *J Burn Care Rehabil* 2005; 26: 33-41.
[89] Oplatek, A; Brown, K; Sen, S, et al. Long-term follow-up of patients treated for toxic epidermal necrolysis. *J Burn Care Res* 2006; 27: 26-33.
[90] Arvidson, J; Kildal, M; Linde, T, et al. Toxic epidermal necrolysis and hemolytic uremic syndrome after allogeneic stem-cell transplantation. *Pediatr Transplant* 2007; 11: 689-693.
[91] Gaultier, F; Rochefort, J; Landru, MM, et al. Severe and unrecognized dental abnormalities after drug-induced epidermal necrolysis. *Arch Dermatol* 2009; 145: 1332-1333.
[92] Quinn, AM; Brown, K; Bonish, BK, et al. Uncovering histologic criteria with prognostic significance in toxic epidermal necrolysis. *Arch Dermatol* 2005; 141: 683-687.
[93] Paquet, P; Paquet, F; Al Saleh, W, et al. Immunoregulatory effector cells in drug-induced toxic epidermal necrolysis. *Am J Dermatopathol* 2000; 22: 413-417.
[94] Paquet, P; Delvenne, P; Piérard, GE. Drug interactions with normal and TEN epidermal keratinocytes. *Curr Drug Saf* 2012; 7: 352-356.
[95] Faye, O; Wechsler, J; Roujeau, JC. Cell-mediated immunologic mechanism and severity of TEN. *Arch Dermatol* 2005; 141: 775-776.
[96] Hermanns-Lê, T; Paquet, P; Piérard-Franchimont, C, et al. Regulatory function of factor-XIIIa-positive dendrocytes in incipient toxic epidermal necrolysis and graft-versus-host reaction. A hypothesis. *Dermatology* 1999; 198: 184-186.
[97] Paquet, P; Quatresooz, P; Piérard, GE. Factor-XIIIa-positive dendrocytes in drug-induced toxic epidermal necrolysis (Lyell's syndrome): paradoxical activation in skin and rarefaction in lymph nodes. *Dermatology* 2003; 206: 374-378.
[98] Verneuil, L; Ratajczak, P; Allabert, C, et al. Endothelial cell apoptosis in severe drug-induced bullous eruptions. *Br J Dermatol* 2009; 161: 1371-1375.
[99] Williams, GP; Mudhar, HS; Leyland, M. Early pathological features of the cornea in toxic epidermal necrolysis. *Br J Ophthalmol* 2007; 91: 1129-1132.
[100] Puangsricharern, V; Tseng, SC. Cytologic evidence of corneal diseases with limbal stem cell deficiency. *Ophthalmology* 1995; 102: 1476-1485.
[101] de Sica-Chapman, A; Williams, G; Soni, N, et al. Granulocyte colony-stimulating factor in toxic epidermal necrolysis (TEN) and Chelsea &

Westminster TEN management protocol. *Br J Dermatol* 2010; 162: 860-865.

[102] Paquet, P; Meuwis, MA; Mazzucchelli, G, et al. Proteomic kinetic analysis of blister fluid and serum in a patient with drug-induced toxic epidermal necrolysis. A comparison with skin immunohistochemistry. *Curr Drug Saf* 2012; 7: 339-351.

[103] Engelhardt, SL; Schurr, MJ; Helgerson, RB. Toxic epidermal necrolysis: an analysis of referral patterns and steroid usage. *J Burn Care Rehabil* 1997; 18: 520-524.

[104] Bachot, N; Roujeau, JC. Differential diagnosis of severe cutaneous drug eruptions. *Am J Clin Dermatol* 2003; 4: 561-572.

[105] Auquier-Dunant, A; Mockenhaupt, M; Naldi, L, et al. Correlations between clinical patterns and causes of erythema multiforme majus, Stevens-Johnson syndrome, and toxic epidermal necrolysis: results of an international prospective study. *Arch Dermatol* 2002; 138: 1019-1024.

[106] Lam, NS; Yang, YH; Wang, LC, et al. Clinical characteristics of childhood erythema multiforme, Stevens-Johnson syndrome and toxic epidermal necrolysis in Taiwanese children. *J Microbiol Immunol Infect* 2004; 37: 366-370.

[107] Quaglino, P; Caproni, M; Osella-Abate, S, et al. Serum interleukin-13 levels are increased in patients with Stevens-Johnson syndrome/ toxic epidermal necrolysis but not in those with erythema multiforme. *Br J Dermatol* 2008; 158: 184-186.

[108] Macedo, FI; Faris, J; Lum, LG, et al. Extensive Toxic Epidermal Necrolysis Versus Acute Graft Versus Host Disease After Allogenic Hematopoietic Stem-Cell Transplantation: Challenges in Diagnosis and Management. *J Burn Care Res* 2014; 35: e431-435.

[109] Takeda, H; Mitsuhashi, Y; Kondo, S, et al. Toxic epidermal necrolysis possibly linked to hyperacute graft-versus-host disease after allogeneic bone marrow transplantation. *J Dermatol* 1997; 24: 635-641.

[110] Stone, N; Sheerin, S; Burge, S. Toxic epidermal necrolysis and graft vs. host disease: a clinical spectrum but a diagnostic dilemma. *Clin Exp Dermatol* 1999; 24: 260-262.

[111] Piérard, GE; Hermanns-Lê, T; Paquet, P, et al. Toxic Epidermal Necrolysis and Graft-versus-Host Reaction: Revisiting a Puzzling Similarity. *ISRN Dermatol* 2013; 2013: 651590.

[112] Whitaker-Menezes, D; Jones, SC; Friedman, TM, et al. An epithelial target site in experimental graft-versus-host disease and cytokine-

mediated cytotoxicity is defined by cytokeratin 15 expression. *Biol Blood Marrow Transplant* 2003; 9: 559-570.

[113] Zhan, Q; Signoretti, S; Whitaker-Menezes, D, et al. Cytokeratin15-positive basal epithelial cells targeted in graft-versus-host disease express a constitutive antiapoptotic phenotype. *J Invest Dermatol* 2007; 127: 106-115.

[114] Hermanns-Lê, T; Paquet, P; Nikkels, AF, et al. Prolonged imiquimod treatment and graft-versus-host reaction: histological mimicry in the skin infiltration pattern of the monocyte-macrophage-dendrocyte lineage. *Dermatology* 2003; 206: 361-365.

[115] Reed, KM; Sober, AJ. Methotrexate-induced necrolysis. *J Am Acad Dermatol* 1983; 8: 677-679.

[116] Gaigl, Z; Seitz, CS; Brocker, EB, et al. Methotrexate-induced toxic epidermal necrolysis-like skin toxicity. *Eur J Dermatol* 2007; 17: 168-169.

[117] Tummino, C; Barlesi, F; Tchouhadjian, C, et al. Severe cutaneous toxicity after pemetrexed as second line treatment for a refractory non small cell lung cancer. *Rev Mal Respir* 2007; 24: 635-638.

[118] Sawada, Y; Kawakami, C; Nakamura, M, et al. Toxic epidermal necrosis-like dermatosis induced by the first course of methotrexate. *Eur J Dermatol* 2009; 19: 397-398.

[119] Primka, EJ, 3rd; Camisa, C. Methotrexate-induced toxic epidermal necrolysis in a patient with psoriasis. *J Am Acad Dermatol* 1997; 36: 815-818.

[120] Hani, N; Casper, C; Groth, W, et al. Stevens-Johnson syndrome-like exanthema secondary to methotrexate histologically simulating acute graft-versus-host disease. *Eur J Dermatol* 2000; 10: 548-550.

[121] Yang, CH; Yang, LJ; Jaing, TH, et al. Toxic epidermal necrolysis following combination of methotrexate and trimethoprim-sulfamethoxazole. *Int J Dermatol* 2000; 39: 621-623.

[122] Cakesen, H; Oner, AF. Toxic epidermal necrolysis in a girl with leukemia receiving methotrexate. *Indian Pediatr* 2001; 38: 426.

[123] Werchniak, AE; Chaffee, S; Dinulos, JG. Methotrexate-induced bullous acral erythema in a child. *J Am Acad Dermatol* 2005; 52: S93-95.

[124] Tezer, H; Kuskonmaz, B; Kara, A, et al. Intravenous immunoglobulin in the treatment of severe methotrexate-induced acral erythema. *J Pediatr Hematol Oncol* 2008; 30: 391-393.

[125] Quatresooz, P; Piérard, GE. Dermal dendrocyte ballooning. *Am J Clin Dermatol* 2006; 7: 391-392.

[126] Dickgreber, NJ; Sorensen, JB; Paz-Ares, LG, et al. Pemetrexed safety and pharmacokinetics in patients with third-space fluid. *Clin Cancer Res* 2010; 16: 2872-2880.

[127] Piérard-Franchimont, C; Quatresooz, P; Reginster, MA, et al. Revisiting cutaneous adverse reactions to pemetrexed. *Oncol Lett* 2001; 2: 769-772.

[128] Sabatiello, M; Willemaers, V; Lesuisse, M, et al. Pemetrexed-induced pityriasis lichenoides-like dermatitis. *J Eur Acad Dermatol Venereol* 2012; 26: 127-129.

[129] Bosch-Barrera, J; Gaztanaga, M; Ceballos, J, et al. Toxic epidermal necrolysis related to pemetrexed and carboplatin with vitamin B12 and folic acid supplementation for advanced non-small cell lung cancer. *Onkologie* 2009; 32: 580-584.

[130] Rousseau, AF; Bargues, L; Le Bever, H, et al. Effect of gamma-hydroxybutyrate on keratinocytes proliferation: a preliminary prospective controlled study in severe burn patients. *International Journal of Critical, Illness and Injury Science* 2014, Epub Apr 9;

[131] Paquet, P; Piérard, GE. Differential pathomechanisms of epidermal necrolytic blistering diseases. *Int J Mol Med* 2002; 10: 695-699.

[132] Sidoroff, A; Halevy, S; Bavinck, JN, et al. Acute generalized exanthematous pustulosis (AGEP)--a clinical reaction pattern. *J Cutan Pathol* 2001; 28: 113-119.

[133] Britschgi, M; Steiner, UC; Schmid, S, et al. T-cell involvement in drug-induced acute generalized exanthematous pustulosis. *J Clin Invest* 2001; 107: 1433-1441.

[134] Schmid, S; Kuechler, PC; Britschgi, M, et al. Acute generalized exanthematous pustulosis: role of cytotoxic T cells in pustule formation. *Am J Pathol* 2002; 161: 2079-2086.

[135] Cho, YT; Lin, JW; Chen, YC, et al. Generalized bullous fixed drug eruption is distinct from Stevens-Johnson syndrome/toxic epidermal necrolysis by immunohistopathological features. *J Am Acad Dermatol* 2014; 70: 539-548.

[136] Sullivan, JR; Shear, NH. The drug hypersensitivity syndrome: what is the pathogenesis? *Arch Dermatol* 2001; 137: 357-364.

[137] Barbaud, A; Waton, J; Herbeth, B, et al. Comparison of cytokine gene polymorphism in drug-induced maculopapular eruption, urticaria and drug reaction with eosinophilia and systemic symptoms (DRESS). *J Eur Acad Dermatol Venereol* 2014; 28: 491-499.

[138] Mandelcorn, R; Shear, NH. Lupus-associated toxic epidermal necrolysis: a novel manifestation of lupus? *J Am Acad Dermatol* 2003; 48: 525-529.

[139] Baker, MG; Cresce, ND; Ameri, M, et al. Systemic lupus erythematosus presenting as stevens-johnson syndrome/toxic epidermal necrolysis. *J Clin Rheumatol* 2014; 20: 167-171.

[140] Su, SC; Chung, WH. Cytotoxic proteins and therapeutic targets in severe cutaneous adverse reactions. *Toxins (Basel)* 2014; 6: 194-210.

[141] Nayak, S; Acharjya, B. Adverse cutaneous drug reaction. *Indian J Dermatol* 2008; 53: 2-8.

[142] Yuan, J; Guo, S; Hall, D, et al. Toxicogenomics of nevirapine-associated cutaneous and hepatic adverse events among populations of African, Asian, and European descent. *AIDS* 2011; 25: 1271-1280.

[143] Sharma, AM; Uetrecht, J. Bioactivation of drugs in the skin: relationship to cutaneous adverse drug reactions. *Drug Metab Rev* 2014; 46: 1-18.

[144] Mockenhaupt, M; Kelly, JP; Kaufman, D, et al. The risk of Stevens-Johnson syndrome and toxic epidermal necrolysis associated with nonsteroidal antiinflammatory drugs: a multinational perspective. *J Rheumatol* 2003; 30: 2234-2240.

[145] La Grenade, L; Lee, L; Weaver, J, et al. Comparison of reporting of Stevens-Johnson syndrome and toxic epidermal necrolysis in association with selective COX-2 inhibitors. *Drug Saf* 2005; 28: 917-924.

[146] Mockenhaupt, M; Messenheimer, J; Tennis, P, et al. Risk of Stevens-Johnson syndrome and toxic epidermal necrolysis in new users of antiepileptics. *Neurology* 2005; 64: 1134-1138.

[147] Halevy, S; Ghislain, PD; Mockenhaupt, M, et al. Allopurinol is the most common cause of Stevens-Johnson syndrome and toxic epidermal necrolysis in Europe and Israel. *J Am Acad Dermatol* 2008; 58: 25-32.

[148] Joao, EC; Calvet, GA; Menezes, JA, et al. Nevirapine toxicity in a cohort of HIV-1-infected pregnant women. *Am J Obstet Gynecol* 2006; 194: 199-202.

[149] Reddy, RB; Shekar, PC; Chandra, KL, et al. Oral lesions associated with Nevirapine-induced Stevens-Johnson syndrome and toxic epidermal necrolysis: A report of 10 cases. *J Oral Maxillofac Pathol* 2013; 17: 431-435.

[150] Mockenhaupt, M; Viboud, C; Dunant, A, et al. Stevens-Johnson syndrome and toxic epidermal necrolysis: assessment of medication risks with emphasis on recently marketed drugs. The EuroSCAR-study. *J Invest Dermatol* 2008; 128: 35-44.

[151] Ball, R; Ball, LK; Wise, RP, et al. Stevens-Johnson syndrome and toxic epidermal necrolysis after vaccination: reports to the vaccine adverse event reporting system. *Pediatr Infect Dis J* 2001; 20: 219-223.

[152] Hilgendorf, I; Casper, J; Sviland, L, et al. Toxic epidermal necrolysis after allogeneic haematopoietic stem cell transplantation. *Bone Marrow Transplant* 2007; 39: 245-246.

[153] Jongen-Lavrencic, M; Schneeberger, PM; van der Hoeven, JG. Ciprofloxacin-induced toxic epidermal necrolysis in a patient with systemic lupus erythematosus. *Infection* 2003; 31: 428-429.

[154] Horne, NS; Narayan, AR; Young, RM, et al. Toxic epidermal necrolysis in systemic lupus erythematosus. *Autoimmun Rev* 2006; 5: 160-164.

[155] Aguiar, D; Pazo, R; Duran, I, et al. Toxic epidermal necrolysis in patients receiving anticonvulsants and cranial irradiation: a risk to consider. *J Neurooncol* 2004; 66: 345-350.

[156] Gravante, G; Delogu, D; Esposito, G, et al. Toxic epidermal necrolysis in oncologic patients. *Am J Clin Dermatol* 2006; 7: 397-398.

[157] Marque, M; Girard, C; Bessis, D, et al. Acute onset Hodgkin's disease following Lyell's syndrome. *Ann Dermatol Venereol* 2007; 134: 767-770.

[158] Saiag, P; Caumes, E; Chosidow, O, et al. Drug-induced toxic epidermal necrolysis (Lyell syndrome) in patients infected with the human immunodeficiency virus. *J Am Acad Dermatol* 1992; 26: 567-574.

[159] Rzany, B; Mockenhaupt, M; Stocker, U, et al. Incidence of Stevens-Johnson syndrome and toxic epidermal necrolysis in patients with the acquired immunodeficiency syndrome in Germany. *Arch Dermatol* 1993; 129: 1059.

[160] Correia, O; Delgado, L; Santos, C, et al. HIV-1 in blister fluid of a patient with toxic epidermal necrolysis and AIDS. *Lancet* 1994; 344: 1432-1433.

[161] Acheampong, EA; Parveen, Z; Muthoga, LW, et al. Molecular interactions of human immunodeficiency virus type 1 with primary human oral keratinocytes. *J Virol* 2005; 79: 8440-8453.

[162] Borgiani, P; Di Fusco, D; Erba, F, et al. HCP5 genetic variant (RS3099844) contributes to Nevirapine-induced Stevens Johnsons Syndrome/Toxic Epidermal Necrolysis susceptibility in a population from Mozambique. *Eur J Clin Pharmacol* 2014; 70: 275-278.

[163] Rotunda, A; Hirsch, RJ; Scheinfeld, N, et al. Severe cutaneous reactions associated with the use of human immunodeficiency virus medications. *Acta Derm Venereol* 2003; 83: 1-9.

[164] Yeung, CK; Ma, SY; Hon, C, et al. Aetiology in sixteen cases of toxic epidermal necrolysis and Stevens-Johnson syndrome admitted within

eight months in a teaching hospital. *Acta Derm Venereol* 2003; 83: 179-182.
[165] Cristallo, AF; Schroeder, J; Citterio, A, et al. A study of HLA class I and class II 4-digit allele level in Stevens-Johnson syndrome and toxic epidermal necrolysis. *Int J Immunogenet* 2011; 38: 303-309.
[166] Bharadwaj, M; Illing, P; Theodossis, A, et al. Drug hypersensitivity and human leukocyte antigens of the major histocompatibility complex. *Annu Rev Pharmacol Toxicol* 2012; 52: 401-431.
[167] Niihara, H; Kakamu, T; Fujita, Y, et al. HLA-A31 strongly associates with carbamazepine-induced adverse drug reactions but not with carbamazepine-induced lymphocyte proliferation in a Japanese population. *J Dermatol* 2012; 39: 594-601.
[168] Pavlos, R; Mallal, S; Ostrov, D, et al. Fever, Rash, and Systemic Symptoms: Understanding the Role of Virus and HLA in Severe Cutaneous Drug Allergy. *J Allergy Clin Immunol Pract* 2014; 2: 21-33.
[169] Borroni, RG. Pharmacogenetic markers of severe cutaneous adverse drug reactions. *G Ital Dermatol Venereol* 2014; 149: 219-226.
[170] Chung, WH; Hung, SI. Recent advances in the genetics and immunology of Stevens-Johnson syndrome and toxic epidermal necrosis. *J Dermatol Sci* 2012; 66: 190-196.
[171] Roychowdhury, S; Vyas, PM; Reilly, TP, et al. Characterization of the formation and localization of sulfamethoxazole and dapsone-associated drug-protein adducts in human epidermal keratinocytes. *J Pharmacol Exp Ther* 2005; 314: 43-52.
[172] Pichler, WJ. Pharmacological interaction of drugs with antigen-specific immune receptors: the p-i concept. *Curr Opin Allergy Clin Immunol* 2002; 2: 301-305.
[173] Gerber, BO; Pichler, WJ. Noncovalent interactions of drugs with immune receptors may mediate drug-induced hypersensitivity reactions. *AAPS J* 2006; 8: E160-165.
[174] Yang, CW; Hung, SI; Juo, CG, et al. HLA-B*1502-bound peptides: implications for the pathogenesis of carbamazepine-induced Stevens-Johnson syndrome. *J Allergy Clin Immunol* 2007; 120: 870-877.
[175] Chung, WH; Hung, SI; Chen, YT. Human leukocyte antigens and drug hypersensitivity. *Curr Opin Allergy Clin Immunol* 2007; 7: 317-323.
[176] Roujeau, JC; Huynh, TN; Bracq, C, et al. Genetic susceptibility to toxic epidermal necrolysis. *Arch Dermatol* 1987; 123: 1171-1173.

[177] Hung, SI; Chung, WH; Jee, SH, et al. Genetic susceptibility to carbamazepine-induced cutaneous adverse drug reactions. *Pharmacogenet Genomics* 2006; 16: 297-306.

[178] Hung, SI; Chung, WH; Liou, LB, et al. HLA-B*5801 allele as a genetic marker for severe cutaneous adverse reactions caused by allopurinol. *Proc Natl Acad Sci U S A* 2005; 102: 4134-4139.

[179] Ueta, M; Sotozono, C; Tokunaga, K, et al. Strong association between HLA-A*0206 and Stevens-Johnson syndrome in the Japanese. *Am J Ophthalmol* 2007; 143: 367-368.

[180] Lonjou, C; Thomas, L; Borot, N, et al. A marker for Stevens-Johnson syndrome ...: ethnicity matters. *Pharmacogenomics J* 2006; 6: 265-268.

[181] Pirmohamed, M; Arbuckle, JB; Bowman, CE, et al. Investigation into the multidimensional genetic basis of drug-induced Stevens-Johnson syndrome and toxic epidermal necrolysis. *Pharmacogenomics* 2007; 8: 1661-1691.

[182] Lonjou, C; Borot, N; Sekula, P, et al. A European study of HLA-B in Stevens-Johnson syndrome and toxic epidermal necrolysis related to five high-risk drugs. *Pharmacogenet Genomics* 2008; 18: 99-107.

[183] Ueta, M; Tokunaga, K; Sotozono, C, et al. HLA class I and II gene polymorphisms in Stevens-Johnson syndrome with ocular complications in Japanese. *Mol Vis* 2008; 14: 550-555.

[184] Dainichi, T; Uchi, H; Moroi, Y, et al. Stevens-Johnson syndrome, drug-induced hypersensitivity syndrome and toxic epidermal necrolysis caused by allopurinol in patients with a common HLA allele: what causes the diversity? *Dermatology* 2007; 215: 86-88.

[185] Ueta, M; Sotozono, C; Inatomi, T, et al. Toll-like receptor 3 gene polymorphisms in Japanese patients with Stevens-Johnson syndrome. *Br J Ophthalmol* 2007; 91: 962-965.

[186] Le Cleach, L; Delaire, S; Boumsell, L, et al. Blister fluid T lymphocytes during toxic epidermal necrolysis are functional cytotoxic cells which express human natural killer (NK) inhibitory receptors. *Clin Exp Immunol* 2000; 119: 225-230.

[187] Yawalkar, N; Egli, F; Hari, Y, et al. Infiltration of cytotoxic T cells in drug-induced cutaneous eruptions. *Clin Exp Allergy* 2000; 30: 847-855.

[188] Pichler, WJ. T cells in drug allergy. *Curr Allergy Asthma Rep* 2002; 2: 9-15.

[189] Nassif, A; Bensussan, A; Boumsell, L, et al. Toxic epidermal necrolysis: effector cells are drug-specific cytotoxic T cells. *J Allergy Clin Immunol* 2004; 114: 1209-1215.

[190] Godfrey, DI; MacDonald, HR; Kronenberg, M, et al. NKT cells: what's in a name? *Nat Rev Immunol* 2004; 4: 231-237.

[191] Teraki, Y; Kawabe, M; Izaki, S. Possible role of TH17 cells in the pathogenesis of Stevens-Johnson syndrome and toxic epidermal necrolysis. *J Allergy Clin Immunol* 2013; 131: 907-909.

[192] Chung, WH; Hung, SI; Yang, JY, et al. Granulysin is a key mediator for disseminated keratinocyte death in Stevens-Johnson syndrome and toxic epidermal necrolysis. *Nat Med* 2008; 14: 1343-1350.

[193] Nagasawa, M; Isoda, T; Itoh, S, et al. Analysis of serum granulysin in patients with hematopoietic stem-cell transplantation: its usefulness as a marker of graft-versus-host reaction. *Am J Hematol* 2006; 81: 340-348.

[194] Nassif, A; Bensussan, A; Dorothee, G, et al. Drug specific cytotoxic T-cells in the skin lesions of a patient with toxic epidermal necrolysis. *J Invest Dermatol* 2002; 118: 728-733.

[195] Trapani, JA; Smyth, MJ. Functional significance of the perforin/granzyme cell death pathway. *Nat Rev Immunol* 2002; 2: 735-747.

[196] Voskoboinik, I; Thia, MC; Fletcher, J, et al. Calcium-dependent plasma membrane binding and cell lysis by perforin are mediated through its C2 domain: A critical role for aspartate residues 429, 435, 483, and 485 but not 491. *J Biol Chem* 2005; 280: 8426-8434.

[197] Law, RH; Lukoyanova, N; Voskoboinik, I, et al. The structural basis for membrane binding and pore formation by lymphocyte perforin. *Nature* 2010; 468: 447-451.

[198] Lord, SJ; Rajotte, RV; Korbutt, GS, et al. Granzyme B: a natural born killer. *Immunol Rev* 2003; 193: 31-38.

[199] Bots, M; Medema, JP. Granzymes at a glance. *J Cell Sci* 2006; 119: 5011-5014.

[200] Bird, CH; Sun, J; Ung, K, et al. Cationic sites on granzyme B contribute to cytotoxicity by promoting its uptake into target cells. *Mol Cell Biol* 2005; 25: 7854-7867.

[201] Veugelers, K; Motyka, B; Goping, IS, et al. Granule-mediated killing by granzyme B and perforin requires a mannose 6-phosphate receptor and is augmented by cell surface heparan sulfate. *Mol Biol Cell* 2006; 17: 623-633.

[202] Keefe, D; Shi, L; Feske, S, et al. Perforin triggers a plasma membrane-repair response that facilitates CTL induction of apoptosis. *Immunity* 2005; 23: 249-262.

[203] Heibein, JA; Goping, IS; Barry, M, et al. Granzyme B-mediated cytochrome c release is regulated by the Bcl-2 family members bid and Bax. *J Exp Med* 2000; 192: 1391-1402.

[204] Sutton, VR; Wowk, ME; Cancilla, M, et al. Caspase activation by granzyme B is indirect, and caspase autoprocessing requires the release of proapoptotic mitochondrial factors. *Immunity* 2003; 18: 319-329.

[205] Goping, IS; Sawchuk, T; Rieger, A, et al. Cytotoxic T lymphocytes overcome Bcl-2 inhibition: target cells contribute to their own demise. *Blood* 2008; 111: 2142-2151.

[206] Paquet, P; De Groote, D; Piérard, GE. Functionally active macrophage-derived myeloperoxidase in the skin of drug-induced toxic epidermal necrolysis. *Dermatology* 2010; 220: 201-207.

[207] Tohyama, M; Watanabe, H; Murakami, S, et al. Possible involvement of CD14+ CD16+ monocyte lineage cells in the epidermal damage of Stevens-Johnson syndrome and toxic epidermal necrolysis. *Br J Dermatol* 2012; 166: 322-330.

[208] Paquet, P; Nusgens, BV; Piérard, GE, et al. Gelatinases in drug-induced toxic epidermal necrolysis. *Eur J Clin Invest* 1998; 28: 528-532.

[209] Moral, A; Palou, J; Lafuente, A, et al. Immunohistochemical study of alpha, mu and pi class glutathione S transferase expression in malignant melanoma. MMM Group. Multidisciplinary Malignant Melanoma Group. *Br J Dermatol* 1997; 136: 345-350.

[210] Paquet, P; Piérard, GE. Glutathione-S-transferase pi expression in toxic epidermal necrolysis: a marker of putative oxidative stress in keratinocytes. *Skin Pharmacol Physiol* 2007; 20: 66-70.

[211] Hayes, JD; Pulford, DJ. The glutathione S-transferase supergene family: regulation of GST and the contribution of the isoenzymes to cancer chemoprotection and drug resistance. *Crit Rev Biochem Mol Biol* 1995; 30: 445-600.

[212] Sarafian, TA; Bredesen, DE. Is apoptosis mediated by reactive oxygen species? *Free Radic Res* 1994; 21: 1-8.

[213] Lange, RW; Hayden, PJ; Chignell, CF, et al. Anthralin stimulates keratinocyte-derived proinflammatory cytokines via generation of reactive oxygen species. *Inflamm Res* 1998; 47: 174-181.

[214] Paquet, P; Ribbens, C; Piérard, GE. Epidermal interleukin-8 and its receptor CXCR2 in drug-induced toxic epidermal necrolysis. *Clin Exp Dermatol* 2007; 32: 728-732.

[215] Herzenberg, LA; De Rosa, SC; Dubs, JG, et al. Glutathione deficiency is associated with impaired survival in HIV disease. *Proc Natl Acad Sci U S A* 1997; 94: 1967-1972.
[216] Korndorfer, IP; Brueckner, F; Skerra, A. The crystal structure of the human (S100A8/S100A9)2 heterotetramer, calprotectin, illustrates how conformational changes of interacting alpha-helices can determine specific association of two EF-hand proteins. *J Mol Biol* 2007; 370: 887-898.
[217] Paquet, P; Piérard, GE. Epidermal calprotectin in drug-induced toxic epidermal necrolysis. *J Cutan Pathol* 1999; 26: 301-305.
[218] Korkiamaki, T; Yla-Outinen, H; Koivunen, J, et al. An intact actin-containing cytoskeleton is required for capacitative calcium entry, but not for ATP-induced calcium-mediated cell signaling in cultured human keratinocytes. *Med Sci Monit* 2003; 9: BR199-207.
[219] Ross, K; Parker, G; Whitaker, M, et al. Inhibition of calcium-independent phospholipase A impairs agonist-induced calcium entry in keratinocytes. *Br J Dermatol* 2008; 158: 31-37.
[220] Trump, BF; Berezesky, IK. The role of altered [Ca2+]i regulation in apoptosis, oncosis, and necrosis. *Biochim Biophys Acta* 1996; 1313: 173-178.
[221] Stahlhut, M; Bertelsen, M; Hoyer-Hansen, M, et al. Ingenol mebutate: induced cell death patterns in normal and cancer epithelial cells. *J Drugs Dermatol* 2012; 11: 1181-1192.
[222] Randhawa, SR; Chahine, BG; Lowery-Nordberg, M, et al. Underexpression and overexpression of Fas and Fas ligand: a double-edged sword. *Ann Allergy Asthma Immunol* 2010; 104: 286-292.
[223] Abe, R; Shimizu, T; Shibaki, A, et al. Toxic epidermal necrolysis and Stevens-Johnson syndrome are induced by soluble Fas ligand. *Am J Pathol* 2003; 162: 1515-1520.
[224] Viard-Leveugle, I; Gaide, O; Jankovic, D, et al. TNF-alpha and IFN-gamma are potential inducers of Fas-mediated keratinocyte apoptosis through activation of inducible nitric oxide synthase in toxic epidermal necrolysis. *J Invest Dermatol* 2013; 133: 489-498.
[225] Murata, J; Abe, R; Shimizu, H. Increased soluble Fas ligand levels in patients with Stevens-Johnson syndrome and toxic epidermal necrolysis preceding skin detachment. *J Allergy Clin Immunol* 2008; 122: 992-1000.

[226] Fu, M; Gao, Y; Pan, Y, et al. Recovered patients with Stevens-Johson syndrome and toxic epidermal necrolysis maintain long-lived IFN-gamma and sFasL memory response. *PLoS One* 2012; 7: e45516.

[227] Viard-Leveugle, I; Bullani, RR; Meda, P, et al. Intracellular localization of keratinocyte Fas ligand explains lack of cytolytic activity under physiological conditions. *J Biol Chem* 2003; 278: 16183-16188.

[228] Xiao, S; Jodo, S; Sung, SS, et al. A novel signaling mechanism for soluble CD95 ligand. Synergy with anti-CD95 monoclonal antibodies for apoptosis and NF-kappaB nuclear translocation. *J Biol Chem* 2002; 277: 50907-50913.

[229] Wilson, NS; Dixit, V; Ashkenazi, A. Death receptor signal transducers: nodes of coordination in immune signaling networks. *Nat Immunol* 2009; 10: 348-355.

[230] Knox, PG; Milner, AE; Green, NK, et al. Inhibition of metalloproteinase cleavage enhances the cytotoxicity of Fas ligand. *J Immunol* 2003; 170: 677-685.

[231] Garcia-Doval, I; Florez, A; De La Torre, C, et al. Transient verrucous hyperplasia after toxic epidermal necrolysis. *Br J Dermatol* 2003; 149: 1082-1083.

[232] Singh, R; Chen, C; Phelps, RG, et al. Stem cells in the skin and their role in oncogenesis. *J Eur Acad Dermatol Venereol* 2014; 28: 542-549.

[233] Abbas, O; Mahalingam, M. Epidermal stem cells: practical perspectives and potential uses. *Br J Dermatol* 2009; 161: 228-236.

[234] Schreder, A; Pierard, GE; Paquet, P, et al. Facing towards epidermal stem cells (Review). *Int J Mol Med* 2010; 26: 171-174.

[235] Jullien, D; Prevot, G; Wolkenstein, P, et al. Eruptive nevus in the course of Lyell syndrome. *Ann Dermatol Venereol* 1995; 122: 540-542.

[236] Paquet, P; Arrese, JE; Greimers, R, et al. Eruptive speckled melanocytic naevi following druinduced toxic epidermal necrolysis. *Eur J Dermatol* 1995; 5: 379-382.

[237] Paquet, P; Jacob, E; Quatresooz, P, et al. Delayed reepithelialization and scarring deregulation following drug-induced toxic epidermal necrolysis. *Burns* 2007; 33: 100-104.

[238] Lehloenya, RJ; Esmail, F; Christians, SJ, et al. Toxic epidermal necrolysis with failure of re-epithelialization. Could umbilical cord mesenchymal stem cell transplantation have a role? *J Eur Acad Dermatol Venereol* 2013; 27: 923-925.

[239] Ito, K; Takigawa, M. Immune privilege and alopecia areata. *Expert Rev Dermatol* 2010; 5: 141-148.

[240] Purba, TS; Haslam, IS; Poblet, E, et al. Human epithelial hair follicle stem cells and their progeny: current state of knowledge, the widening gap in translational research and future challenges. *Bioessays* 2014; 36: 513-525.

[241] Ruckert, R; Lindner, G; Bulfone-Paus, S, et al. High-dose proinflammatory cytokines induce apoptosis of hair bulb keratinocytes in vivo. *Br J Dermatol* 2000; 143: 1036-1039.

[242] Arnold, R; Seifert, M; Asadullah, K, et al. Crosstalk between keratinocytes and T lymphocytes via Fas/Fas ligand interaction: modulation by cytokines. *J Immunol* 1999; 162: 7140-7147.

[243] Seitz, CS; Freiberg, RA; Hinata, K, et al. NF-kappaB determines localization and features of cell death in epidermis. *J Clin Invest* 2000; 105: 253-260.

[244] Liu, ZG. Molecular mechanism of TNF signaling and beyond. *Cell Res* 2005; 15: 24-27.

[245] Norman, MU; Lister, KJ; Yang, YH, et al. TNF regulates leukocyte-endothelial cell interactions and microvascular dysfunction during immune complex-mediated inflammation. *Br J Pharmacol* 2005; 144: 265-274.

[246] Kelly, M; Hwang, JM; Kubes, P. Modulating leukocyte recruitment in inflammation. *J Allergy Clin Immunol* 2007; 120: 3-10.

[247] Caproni, M; Torchia, D; Schincaglia, E, et al. Expression of cytokines and chemokine receptors in the cutaneous lesions of erythema multiforme and Stevens-Johnson syndrome/toxic epidermal necrolysis. *Br J Dermatol* 2006; 155: 722-728.

[248] Schroder, K; Hertzog, PJ; Ravasi, T, et al. Interferon-gamma: an overview of signals, mechanisms and functions. *J Leukoc Biol* 2004; 75: 163-189.

[249] Nassif, A; Moslehi, H; Le Gouvello, S, et al. Evaluation of the potential role of cytokines in toxic epidermal necrolysis. *J Invest Dermatol* 2004; 123: 850-855.

[250] Paul, C; Wolkenstein, P; Adle, H, et al. Apoptosis as a mechanism of keratinocyte death in toxic epidermal necrolysis. *Br J Dermatol* 1996; 134: 710-714.

[251] Paquet, P; Piérard, GE. Toxic epidermal necrolysis: revisiting the tentative link between early apoptosis and late necrosis (review). *Int J Mol Med* 2007; 19: 3-10.

[252] Li, J; Yuan, J. Caspases in apoptosis and beyond. *Oncogene* 2008; 27: 6194-6206.

[253] Green, DR; Reed, JC. Mitochondria and apoptosis. *Science* 1998; 281: 1309-1312.

[254] Correia, O; Delgado, L; Barbosa, IL, et al. Increased interleukin 10, tumor necrosis factor alpha, and interleukin 6 levels in blister fluid of toxic epidermal necrolysis. *J Am Acad Dermatol* 2002; 47: 58-62.

[255] Lerner, LH; Qureshi, AA; Reddy, BV, et al. Nitric oxide synthase in toxic epidermal necrolysis and Stevens-Johnson syndrome. *J Invest Dermatol* 2000; 114: 196-199.

[256] Marzano, AV; Frezzolini, A; Caproni, M, et al. Immunohistochemical expression of apoptotic markers in drug-induced erythema multiforme, Stevens-Johnson syndrome and toxic epidermal necrolysis. *Int J Immunopathol Pharmacol* 2007; 20: 557-566.

[257] Williams, GP; Tomlins, PJ; Denniston, AK, et al. Elevation of conjunctival epithelial CD45INTCD11b(+)CD16(+)CD14(-) neutrophils in ocular Stevens-Johnson syndrome and toxic epidermal necrolysis. *Invest Ophthalmol Vis Sci* 2013; 54: 4578-4585.

[258] Tapia, B; Padial, A; Sanchez-Sabate, E, et al. Involvement of CCL27-CCR10 interactions in drug-induced cutaneous reactions. *J Allergy Clin Immunol* 2004; 114: 335-340.

[259] Leyva, L; Torres, MJ; Posadas, S, et al. Anticonvulsant-induced toxic epidermal necrolysis: monitoring the immunologic response. *J Allergy Clin Immunol* 2000; 105: 157-165.

[260] Mayorga, C; Torres, MJ; Corzo, JL, et al. Improvement of toxic epidermal necrolysis after the early administration of a single high dose of intravenous immunoglobulin. *Ann Allergy Asthma Immunol* 2003; 91: 86-91.

[261] Segura Huerta, AA; Tordera, P; Cercos, AC, et al. Toxic epidermal necrolysis associated with interleukin-2. *Ann Pharmacother* 2002; 36: 1171-1174.

[262] Inachi, S; Mizutani, H; Shimizu, M. Epidermal apoptotic cell death in erythema multiforme and Stevens-Johnson syndrome. Contribution of perforin-positive cell infiltration. *Arch Dermatol* 1997; 133: 845-849.

[263] Mingari, MC; Ponte, M; Bertone, S, et al. HLA class I-specific inhibitory receptors in human T lymphocytes: interleukin 15-induced expression of CD94/NKG2A in superantigen- or alloantigen-activated CD8+ T cells. *Proc Natl Acad Sci U S A* 1998; 95: 1172-1177.

[264] Caproni, M; Torchia, D; Schincaglia, E, et al. The CD40/CD40 ligand system is expressed in the cutaneous lesions of erythema multiforme and

Stevens-Johnson syndrome/toxic epidermal necrolysis spectrum. *Br J Dermatol* 2006; 154: 319-324.
[265] Ettorre, A; Andreassi, M; Anselmi, C, et al. Involvement of oxidative stress in apoptosis induced by a mixture of isothiazolinones in normal human keratinocytes. *J Invest Dermatol* 2003; 121: 328-336.
[266] Armeni, T; Battino, M; Stronati, A, et al. Total antioxidant capacity and nuclear DNA damage in keratinocytes after exposure to H2O2. *Biol Chem* 2001; 382: 1697-1705.
[267] Glasser, DL; Burroughs, SH. Valdecoxib-induced toxic epidermal necrolysis in a patient allergic to sulfa drugs. *Pharmacotherapy* 2003; 23: 551-553.
[268] Huang, LY; Liao, WC; Chiou, CC, et al. Fatal toxic epidermal necrolysis induced by carbamazepine treatment in a patient who previously had carbamazepine-induced Stevens-Johnson syndrome. *J Formos Med Assoc* 2007; 106: 1032-1037.
[269] Pasricha, JS; Khaitan, BK; Shantharaman, R, et al. Toxic epidermal necrolysis. *Int J Dermatol* 1996; 35: 523-527.
[270] de Araujo, E; Dessirier, V; Lapree, G, et al. Death ligand TRAIL, secreted by CD1a+ and CD14+ cells in blister fluids, is involved in killing keratinocytes in toxic epidermal necrolysis. *Exp Dermatol* 2011; 20: 107-112.
[271] Piérard, GE; Uhoda, E. Skin photophysics and colors. *Rev Med Liege* 2005; 60 Suppl 1: 48-52.
[272] Hermanns, JF; Piérard, GE. High-resolution epiluminescence colorimetry of striae distensae. *J Eur Acad Dermatol Venereol* 2006; 20: 282-287.
[273] Devillers, C; Piérard-Franchimont, C; Schreder, A, et al. High resolution skin colorimetry, strain mapping and mechanobiology. *Int J Cosmet Sci* 2010; 32: 241-245.
[274] Wilkins, AJ; Nimmo-Smith, I; Jansons, JE. Colorimeter for the intuitive manipulation of hue and saturation and its role in the study of perceptual distortion. *Ophthalmic Physiol Opt* 1992; 12: 381-385.
[275] Petit, L; Fogouang, L; Uhoda, I, et al. Regional variability in mottled subclinical melanoderma in the elderly. *Exp Gerontol* 2003; 38: 327-331.
[276] Xhauflaire-Uhoda, E; Piérard-Franchimont, C; Piérard, GE, et al. Weathering of the hairless scalp: a study using skin capacitance imaging and ultraviolet light-enhanced visualization. *Clin Exp Dermatol* 2010; 35: 83-85.

[277] Hermanns-Lê, T; Piérard-Franchimont, C; Piérard, GE. Scrutinizing skinfield melanin patterns in young Caucasian women. *Expert Opin Med Diagn* 2013; 7: 455-462.
[278] Lévêque, JL; Xhauflaire-Uhoda, E; Piérard, GE. Skin capacitance imaging, a new technique for investigating the skin surface. *Eur J Dermatol* 2006; 16: 500-506.
[279] Xhauflaire-Uhoda, E; Piérard, GE; Quatresooz, P. The skin landscape following nonoptical capacitance imaging. *Am J Clin Dermatol* 2010; 11: 89-94.
[280] Delvenne, M; Piérard-Franchimont, C; Seidel, L, et al. The weather-beaten dorsal hand clinical rating, shadow casting optical profilometry, and skin capacitance mapping. *Biomed Res Int* 2013; 2013: 913646.
[281] Piérard, GE. In vivo confocal microscopy: a new paradigm in dermatology. *Dermatology* 1993; 186: 4-5.
[282] Corcuff, P; Gonnord, G; Piérard, GE, et al. In vivo confocal microscopy of human skin: a new design for cosmetology and dermatology. *Scanning* 1996; 18: 351-355.
[283] Moscarella, E; Argenziano, G; Lallas, A, et al. Confocal microscopy: a new era in understanding the pathophysiologic background of inflammatory skin diseases. *Exp Dermatol* 2014; 23: 320-321.
[284] Vera, LS; Gueudry, J; Delcampe, A, et al. In vivo confocal microscopic evaluation of corneal changes in chronic Stevens-Johnson syndrome and toxic epidermal necrolysis. *Cornea* 2009; 28: 401-407.
[285] Chen, P; Lin, JJ; Lu, CS, et al. Carbamazepine-induced toxic effects and HLA-B*1502 screening in Taiwan. *N Engl J Med* 2011; 364: 1126-1133.
[286] Wu, K; Reynolds, NJ. Pharmacogenetic screening to prevent carbamazepine-induced toxic epidermal necrolysis and Stevens-Johnson syndrome: a critical appraisal. *Br J Dermatol* 2012; 166: 7-11; discussion 11-14.
[287] Su, SC; Chung, WH. Update on pathobiology in Stevens-Johnson syndrome and toxic epidermal necrolysis. *Dermatol Sin* 2013; 31: 175-180.
[288] Toh, DS; Tan, LL; Aw, DC, et al. Building pharmacogenetics into a pharmacovigilance program in Singapore: using serious skin rash as a pilot study. *Pharmacogenomics J* 2014; 14: 316-321.
[289] Azukizawa, H; Sano, S; Kosaka, H, et al. Prevention of toxic epidermal necrolysis by regulatory T cells. *Eur J Immunol* 2005; 35: 1722-1730.

[290] Eliaszewicz, M; Flahault, A; Roujeau, JC, et al. Prospective evaluation of risk factors of cutaneous drug reactions to sulfonamides in patients with AIDS. *J Am Acad Dermatol* 2002; 47: 40-46.
[291] Abo, T. Extrathymic pathways of T-cell differentiation and immunomodulation. *Int Immunopharmacol* 2001; 1: 1261-1273.
[292] Paquet, P; Jacob, E; Damas, P, et al. Recurrent fatal drug-induced toxic epidermal necrolysis (Lyell's syndrome) after putative beta-lactam cross-reactivity: Case report and scrutiny of antibiotic imputability. *Crit Care Med* 2002; 30: 2580-2583.
[293] Dorafshar, AH; Dickie, SR; Cohn, AB, et al. Antishear therapy for toxic epidermal necrolysis: an alternative treatment approach. *Plast Reconstr Surg* 2008; 122: 154-160.
[294] Bastuji-Garin, S; Fouchard, N; Bertocchi, M, et al. SCORTEN: a severity-of-illness score for toxic epidermal necrolysis. *J Invest Dermatol* 2000; 115: 149-153.
[295] Trent, JT; Kirsner, RS; Romanelli, P, et al. Use of SCORTEN to accurately predict mortality in patients with toxic epidermal necrolysis in the United States. *Arch Dermatol* 2004; 140: 890-892.
[296] Guégan, S; Bastuji-Garin, S; Poszepczynska-Guigne, E, et al. Performance of the SCORTEN during the first five days of hospitalization to predict the prognosis of epidermal necrolysis. *J Invest Dermatol* 2006; 126: 272-276.
[297] Imahara, SD; Holmes, JHt; Heimbach, DM, et al. SCORTEN overestimates mortality in the setting of a standardized treatment protocol. *J Burn Care Res* 2006; 27: 270-275.
[298] Cartotto, R; Mayich, M; Nickerson, D, et al. SCORTEN accurately predicts mortality among toxic epidermal necrolysis patients treated in a burn center. *J Burn Care Res* 2008; 29: 141-146.
[299] Vaishampayan, SS; Das, AL; Verma, R. SCORTEN: does it need modification? *Indian J Dermatol Venereol Leprol* 2008; 74: 35-37.
[300] Sekula, P; Liss, Y; Davidovici, B, et al. Evaluation of SCORTEN on a cohort of patients with Stevens-Johnson syndrome and toxic epidermal necrolysis included in the RegiSCAR study. *J Burn Care Res* 2011; 32: 237-245.
[301] Sassolas, B; Haddad, C; Mockenhaupt, M, et al. ALDEN, an algorithm for assessment of drug causality in Stevens-Johnson Syndrome and toxic epidermal necrolysis: comparison with case-control analysis. *Clin Pharmacol Ther* 2010; 88: 60-68.

[302] Paquet, P; Jennes, S; Rousseau, AF, et al. Effect of N-acetylcysteine combined with infliximab on toxic epidermal necrolysis. A proof-of-concept study. *Burns* 2014; 40: 1707-1712.

[303] Namdar, T; von Wild, T; Siemers, F, et al. Does hypernatremia impact mortality in Toxic Epidermal Necrolysis? *Ger Med Sci* 2010; 8: Doc30.

[304] Trent, JT; Kirsner, RS; Romanelli, P, et al. Analysis of intravenous immunoglobulin for the treatment of toxic epidermal necrolysis using SCORTEN: The University of Miami Experience. *Arch Dermatol* 2003; 139: 39-43.

[305] Knight, L; Muloiwa, R; Dlamini, S, et al. Factors Associated with Increased Mortality in a Predominantly HIV-Infected Population with Stevens Johnson Syndrome and Toxic Epidermal Necrolysis. *PLoS One* 2014; 9: e93543.

[306] Hettiaratchy, S; Moloney, D; Clarke, J. Patients with acute skin loss: are they best managed on a burns unit? *Ann R Coll Surg Engl* 2001; 83: 26-29.

[307] Palmieri, TL; Greenhalgh, DG; Saffle, JR, et al. A multicenter review of toxic epidermal necrolysis treated in U.S. burn centers at the end of the twentieth century. *J Burn Care Rehabil* 2002; 23: 87-96.

[308] Gerdts, B; Vloemans, AF; Kreis, RW. Toxic epidermal necrolysis: 15 years' experience in a Dutch burns centre. *J Eur Acad Dermatol Venereol* 2007; 21: 781-788.

[309] Firoz, BF; Henning, JS; Zarzabal, LA, et al. Toxic epidermal necrolysis: five years of treatment experience from a burn unit. *J Am Acad Dermatol* 2012; 67: 630-635.

[310] Jennes, S; Pierard, GE; Paquet, P. Deciphering supportive treatment strategies for toxic epidermal necrolysis. *Curr Drug Saf* 2012; 7: 361-366.

[311] Garcia-Doval, I; LeCleach, L; Bocquet, H, et al. Toxic epidermal necrolysis and Stevens-Johnson syndrome: does early withdrawal of causative drugs decrease the risk of death? *Arch Dermatol* 2000; 136: 323-327.

[312] Paquet, P; Schaaf-Lafontaine, N; Piérard, GE. Toxic epidermal necrolysis following clindamycin treatment. *Br J Dermatol* 1995; 132: 665-666.

[313] Kano, Y; Hirahara, K; Mitsuyama, Y, et al. Utility of the lymphocyte transformation test in the diagnosis of drug sensitivity: dependence on its timing and the type of drug eruption. *Allergy* 2007; 62: 1439-1444.

[314] Tang, YH; Mockenhaupt, M; Henry, A, et al. Poor relevance of a lymphocyte proliferation assay in lamotrigine-induced Stevens-Johnson syndrome or toxic epidermal necrolysis. *Clin Exp Allergy* 2012; 42: 248-254.

[315] Porebski, G; Pecaric-Petkovic, T; Groux-Keller, M, et al. In vitro drug causality assessment in Stevens-Johnson syndrome - alternatives for lymphocyte transformation test. *Clin Exp Allergy* 2013; 43: 1027-1037.

[316] Windle, EM. Immune modulating nutrition support for a patient with severe toxic epidermal necrolysis. *J Hum Nutr Diet* 2005; 18: 311-314.

[317] Coss-Bu, JA; Jefferson, LS; Levy, ML, et al. Nutrition requirements in patients with toxic epidermal necrolysis. *Nutr Clin Pract* 1997; 12: 81-84.

[318] Mayes, T; Gottschlich, M; Khoury, J, et al. Energy requirements of pediatric patients with Stevens-Johnson syndrome and toxic epidermal necrolysis. *Nutr Clin Pract* 2008; 23: 547-550.

[319] van den Berghe, G; Wouters, P; Weekers, F, et al. Intensive insulin therapy in critically ill patients. *N Engl J Med* 2001; 345: 1359-1367.

[320] Tseng, SC. Acute management of Stevens-Johnson syndrome and toxic epidermal necrolysis to minimize ocular sequelae. *Am J Ophthalmol* 2009; 147: 949-951.

[321] Gregory, DG. The ophthalmologic management of acute Stevens-Johnson syndrome. *Ocul Surf* 2008; 6: 87-95.

[322] Tougeron-Brousseau, B; Delcampe, A; Gueudry, J, et al. Vision-related function after scleral lens fitting in ocular complications of Stevens-Johnson syndrome and toxic epidermal necrolysis. *Am J Ophthalmol* 2009; 148: 852-859 e852.

[323] McGee, T; Munster, A. Toxic epidermal necrolysis syndrome: mortality rate reduced with early referral to regional burn center. *Plast Reconstr Surg* 1998; 102: 1018-1022.

[324] Timsit, JF; Mion, G; Rouyer, N, et al. Bronchopulmonary distress associated with toxic epidermal necrolysis. *Intensive Care Med* 1992; 18: 42-44.

[325] Paquet, P; Pierard, GE. Topical treatment options for drug-induced toxic epidermal necrolysis (TEN). *Expert Opin Pharmacother* 2010; 11: 2447-2458.

[326] Dillon, CK; Lloyd, MS; Dzeiwulski, P. Accurate debridement of toxic epidermal necrolysis using Versajet®. *Burns* 2010; 36: 581-584.

[327] Pianigiani, E; Lerardi, F; Taddeucci, P, et al. Skin allograft in the treatment of toxic epidermal necrolysis (TEN). *Dermatol Surg* 2002; 28: 1173-1176.
[328] Kobayashi, A; Yoshita, T; Sugiyama, K, et al. Amniotic membrane transplantation in acute phase of toxic epidermal necrolysis with severe corneal involvement. *Ophthalmology* 2006; 113: 126-132.
[329] Shay, E; Kheirkhah, A; Liang, L, et al. Amniotic membrane transplantation as a new therapy for the acute ocular manifestations of Stevens-Johnson syndrome and toxic epidermal necrolysis. *Surv Ophthalmol* 2009; 54: 686-696.
[330] Gregory, DG. Treatment of acute Stevens-Johnson syndrome and toxic epidermal necrolysis using amniotic membrane: a review of 10 consecutive cases. *Ophthalmology* 2011; 118: 908-914.
[331] Bhattacharya, S; Tripathi, HN; Gupta, V, et al. Collagen sheet dressings for cutaneous lesions of toxic epidermal necrolysis. *Indian J Plast Surg* 2011; 44: 474-477.
[332] Bannasch, H; Kontny, U; Kruger, M, et al. A semisynthetic bilaminar skin substitute used to treat pediatric full-body toxic epidermal necrolysis: wraparound technique in a 17-month-old girl. *Arch Dermatol* 2004; 140: 160-162.
[333] Huang, S; Fu, X. Tissue-engineered skin: bottleneck or breakthrough. *Int J Burns Trauma* 2011; 1: 1-10.
[334] Li, X; Wang, D; Lu, Z, et al. Umbilical cord mesenchymal stem cell transplantation in drug-induced Stevens-Johnson syndrome. *J Eur Acad Dermatol Venereol* 2013; 27: 659-661.
[335] Arevalo, JM; Lorente, JA. Skin coverage with Biobrane biomaterial for the treatment of patients with toxic epidermal necrolysis. *J Burn Care Rehabil* 1999; 20: 406-410.
[336] Whitaker, IS; Prowse, S; Potokar, TS. A critical evaluation of the use of Biobrane as a biologic skin substitute: a versatile tool for the plastic and reconstructive surgeon. *Ann Plast Surg* 2008; 60: 333-337.
[337] Lindford, AJ; Kaartinen, IS; Virolainen, S, et al. Comparison of Suprathel(R) and allograft skin in the treatment of a severe case of toxic epidermal necrolysis. *Burns* 2011; 37: e67-72.
[338] Pfurtscheller, K; Zobel, G; Roedl, S, et al. Use of Suprathel dressing in a young infant with TEN. *Pediatr Dermatol* 2008; 25: 541-543.
[339] Asz, J; Asz, D; Moushey, R, et al. Treatment of toxic epidermal necrolysis in a pediatric patient with a nanocrystalline silver dressing. *J Pediatr Surg* 2006; 41: e9-12.

[340] Huang, SH; Wu, SH; Sun, IF, et al. AQUACEL Ag in the treatment of toxic epidermal necrolysis (TEN). *Burns* 2008; 34: 63-66.
[341] Smith, SD; Dodds, A; Dixit, S, et al. Role of nanocrystalline silver dressings in the management of toxic epidermal necrolysis (TEN) and TEN/Stevens-Johnson syndrome overlap. *Australas J Dermatol* 2014;
[342] Ng, RW; Cheng, YL. Calcium alginate dressing-related hypercalcemia. *J Burn Care Res* 2007; 28: 203-204.
[343] Lehrer-Bell, KA; Kirsner, RS; Tallman, PG, et al. Treatment of the cutaneous involvement in Stevens-Johnson syndrome and toxic epidermal necrolysis with silver nitrate-impregnated dressings. *Arch Dermatol* 1998; 134: 877-879.
[344] Fumal, I; Braham, C; Paquet, P, et al. The beneficial toxicity paradox of antimicrobials in leg ulcer healing impaired by a polymicrobial flora: a proof-of-concept study. *Dermatology* 2002; 204 Suppl 1: 70-74.
[345] Timsit, JF; Mion, G; Le Gulluche, Y, et al. Severe hypothermia occurring during the course of toxic epidermal necrolysis in patients treated with air-fluidized beds. *Arch Dermatol* 1991; 127: 739-740.
[346] Boorboor, P; Vogt, PM; Bechara, FG, et al. Toxic epidermal necrolysis: use of Biobrane or skin coverage reduces pain, improves mobilisation and decreases infection in elderly patients. *Burns* 2008; 34: 487-492.
[347] Hii, BW; Mahar, PD; Wasiak, J, et al. Hospital management and clinical factors associated with ophthalmic involvement in toxic epidermal necrolysis. *Burns* 2014; 40: 903-908.
[348] Lopez-Garcia, JS; Rivas, L; Garcia-Lozano, I, et al. Amniotic membrane transplantation in acute toxic epidermal necrolysis: histopathologic changes and ocular surface features after 1-year follow-up. *Eur J Ophthalmol* 2014; 24: 667-675.
[349] John, T; Foulks, GN; John, ME, et al. Amniotic membrane in the surgical management of acute toxic epidermal necrolysis. *Ophthalmology* 2002; 109: 351-360.
[350] Tandon, A; Cackett, P; Mulvihill, A, et al. Amniotic membrane grafting for conjunctival and lid surface disease in the acute phase of toxic epidermal necrolysis. *J AAPOS* 2007; 11: 612-613.
[351] Shay, E; Khadem, JJ; Tseng, SC. Efficacy and limitation of sutureless amniotic membrane transplantation for acute toxic epidermal necrolysis. *Cornea* 2010; 29: 359-361.
[352] Ciralsky, JB; Sippel, KC; Gregory, DG. Current ophthalmologic treatment strategies for acute and chronic Stevens-Johnson syndrome

and toxic epidermal necrolysis. *Curr Opin Ophthalmol* 2013; 24: 321-328.

[353] Iyer, G; Srinivasan, B; Agarwal, S, et al. Comprehensive approach to ocular consequences of Stevens Johnson Syndrome - the aftermath of a systemic condition. *Graefes Arch Clin Exp Ophthalmol* 2014; 252: 457-467.

[354] Shammas, MC; Lai, EC; Sarkar, JS, et al. Management of acute Stevens-Johnson syndrome and toxic epidermal necrolysis utilizing amniotic membrane and topical corticosteroids. *Am J Ophthalmol* 2010; 149: 203-213 e202.

[355] Sachdev, R; Bansal, S; Sinha, R, et al. Bilateral microbial keratitis in highly active antiretroviral therapy-induced Stevens-Johnson syndrome and toxic epidermal necrolysis: a case series. *Ocul Immunol Inflamm* 2011; 19: 343-345.

[356] Tomlins, PJ; Parulekar, MV; Rauz, S. "Triple-TEN" in the treatment of acute ocular complications from toxic epidermal necrolysis. *Cornea* 2013; 32: 365-369.

[357] Spies, M; Sanford, AP; Aili Low, JF, et al. Treatment of extensive toxic epidermal necrolysis in children. *Pediatrics* 2001; 108: 1162-1168.

[358] Paquet, P; Piérard, GE; Quatresooz, P. Novel treatments for drug-induced toxic epidermal necrolysis (Lyell's syndrome). *Int Arch Allergy Immunol* 2005; 136: 205-216.

[359] Fromowitz, JS; Ramos-Caro, FA; Flowers, FP. Practical guidelines for the management of toxic epidermal necrolysis and Stevens-Johnson syndrome. *Int J Dermatol* 2007; 46: 1092-1094.

[360] Marchal, G; Bilski-Pasquier, G; Flandrin, G. On a Severe Type of Pluri-Orificial Ectodermosis. Rapidly Favorable Course Due to Corticotherapy. *Bull Mem Soc Med Hop Paris* 1964; 115: 717-720.

[361] van der Meer, JB; Schuttelaar, ML; Toth, GG, et al. Successful dexamethasone pulse therapy in a toxic epidermal necrolysis (TEN) patient featuring recurrent TEN to oxazepam. *Clin Exp Dermatol* 2001; 26: 654-656.

[362] Kardaun, SH; Jonkman, MF. Dexamethasone pulse therapy for Stevens-Johnson syndrome/toxic epidermal necrolysis. *Acta Derm Venereol* 2007; 87: 144-148.

[363] Araki, Y; Sotozono, C; Inatomi, T, et al. Successful treatment of Stevens-Johnson syndrome with steroid pulse therapy at disease onset. *Am J Ophthalmol* 2009; 147: 1004-1011, 1011 e1001.

[364] Viard, I; Wehrli, P; Bullani, R, et al. Inhibition of toxic epidermal necrolysis by blockade of CD95 with human intravenous immunoglobulin. *Science* 1998; 282: 490-493.
[365] Ito, K; Hara, H; Okada, T, et al. Toxic epidermal necrolysis treated with low-dose intravenous immunoglobulin: immunohistochemical study of Fas and Fas-ligand expression. *Clin Exp Dermatol* 2004; 29: 679-680.
[366] Paquet, P; Kaveri, S; Jacob, E, et al. Skin immunoglobulin deposition following intravenous immunoglobulin therapy in toxic epidermal necrolysis. *Exp Dermatol* 2006; 15: 381-386.
[367] Paquet, P; Jacob, E; Damas, P, et al. Treatment of drug-induced toxic epidermal necrolysis (Lyell's syndrome) with intravenous human immunoglobulins. *Burns* 2001; 27: 652-655.
[368] Tristani-Firouzi, P; Petersen, MJ; Saffle, JR, et al. Treatment of toxic epidermal necrolysis with intravenous immunoglobulin in children. *J Am Acad Dermatol* 2002; 47: 548-552.
[369] Bachot, N; Revuz, J; Roujeau, JC. Intravenous immunoglobulin treatment for Stevens-Johnson syndrome and toxic epidermal necrolysis: a prospective noncomparative study showing no benefit on mortality or progression. *Arch Dermatol* 2003; 139: 33-36.
[370] Brown, KM; Silver, GM; Halerz, M, et al. Toxic epidermal necrolysis: does immunoglobulin make a difference? *J Burn Care Rehabil* 2004; 25: 81-88.
[371] Shortt, R; Gomez, M; Mittman, N, et al. Intravenous immunoglobulin does not improve outcome in toxic epidermal necrolysis. *J Burn Care Rehabil* 2004; 25: 246-255.
[372] Faye, O; Roujeau, JC. Treatment of epidermal necrolysis with high-dose intravenous immunoglobulins (IV Ig): clinical experience to date. *Drugs* 2005; 65: 2085-2090.
[373] Tan, AW; Thong, BY; Yip, LW, et al. High-dose intravenous immunoglobulins in the treatment of toxic epidermal necrolysis: an Asian series. *J Dermatol* 2005; 32: 1-6.
[374] French, LE; Trent, JT; Kerdel, FA. Use of intravenous immunoglobulin in toxic epidermal necrolysis and Stevens-Johnson syndrome: our current understanding. *Int Immunopharmacol* 2006; 6: 543-549.
[375] Mittmann, N; Chan, B; Knowles, S, et al. Intravenous immunoglobulin use in patients with toxic epidermal necrolysis and Stevens-Johnson syndrome. *Am J Clin Dermatol* 2006; 7: 359-368.
[376] Stella, M; Clemente, A; Bollero, D, et al. Toxic epidermal necrolysis (TEN) and Stevens-Johnson syndrome (SJS): experience with high-dose

intravenous immunoglobulins and topical conservative approach. A retrospective analysis. *Burns* 2007; 33: 452-459.

[377] Huang, YC; Li, YC; Chen, TJ. The efficacy of intravenous immunoglobulin for the treatment of toxic epidermal necrolysis: a systematic review and meta-analysis. *Br J Dermatol* 2012; 167: 424-432.

[378] Yip, LW; Thong, BY; Tan, AW, et al. High-dose intravenous immunoglobulin in the treatment of toxic epidermal necrolysis: a study of ocular benefits. *Eye (Lond)* 2005; 19: 846-853.

[379] Paquet, P; Piérard, GE. Would cyclosporin A be beneficial to mitigate drug-induced toxic epidermal necrolysis? *Dermatology* 1999; 198: 198-202.

[380] Arevalo, JM; Lorente, JA; Gonzalez-Herrada, C, et al. Treatment of toxic epidermal necrolysis with cyclosporin A. *J Trauma* 2000; 48: 473-478.

[381] Hashim, N; Bandara, D; Tan, E, et al. Early cyclosporine treatment of incipient toxic epidermal necrolysis induced by concomitant use of lamotrigine and sodium valproate. *Acta Derm Venereol* 2004; 84: 90-91.

[382] Valeyrie-Allanore, L; Wolkenstein, P; Brochard, L, et al. Open trial of ciclosporin treatment for Stevens-Johnson syndrome and toxic epidermal necrolysis. *Br J Dermatol* 2010; 163: 847-853.

[383] Danby, FW. Ciclosporin use in toxic epidermal necrolysis. *Br J Dermatol* 2007; 156: 390-391.

[384] Paquet, P; Jacob, E; Damas, P, et al. Analytical quantification of the inflammatory cell infiltrate and CD95R expression during treatment of drug-induced toxic epidermal necrolysis. *Arch Dermatol Res* 2005; 297: 266-273.

[385] Paquet, P; Arrese Estrada, J; Piérard, GE. Oral cyclosporin and alopecia areata. *Dermatology* 1992; 185: 314-315.

[386] Fischer, M; Fiedler, E; Marsch, WC, et al. Antitumour necrosis factor-alpha antibodies (infliximab) in the treatment of a patient with toxic epidermal necrolysis. *Br J Dermatol* 2002; 146: 707-709.

[387] Al-Shouli, S; Abouchala, N; Bogusz, MJ, et al. Toxic epidermal necrolysis associated with high intake of sildenafil and its response to infliximab. *Acta Derm Venereol* 2005; 85: 534-535.

[388] Hunger, RE; Hunziker, T; Buettiker, U, et al. Rapid resolution of toxic epidermal necrolysis with anti-TNF-alpha treatment. *J Allergy Clin Immunol* 2005; 116: 923-924.

[389] Meiss, F; Helmbold, P; Meykadeh, N, et al. Overlap of acute generalized exanthematous pustulosis and toxic epidermal necrolysis: response to antitumour necrosis factor-alpha antibody infliximab: report of three cases. *J Eur Acad Dermatol Venereol* 2007; 21: 717-719.
[390] Famularo, G; Di Dona, B; Canzona, F, et al. Etanercept for toxic epidermal necrolysis. *Ann Pharmacother* 2007; 41: 1083-1084.
[391] Wolkenstein, P; Latarjet, J; Roujeau, JC, et al. Randomised comparison of thalidomide versus placebo in toxic epidermal necrolysis. *Lancet* 1998; 352: 1586-1589.
[392] Velez, A; Moreno, JC. Toxic epidermal necrolysis treated with N-acetylcysteine. *J Am Acad Dermatol* 2002; 46: 469-470.
[393] Redondo, P; de Felipe, I; de la Pena, A, et al. Drug-induced hypersensitivity syndrome and toxic epidermal necrolysis. Treatment with N-acetylcysteine. *Br J Dermatol* 1997; 136: 645-646.
[394] Yavuz, H; Emiroglu, M. Toxic epidermal necrolysis treated with N-acetylcysteine. *Pediatr Int* 2014; 56: e52-54.
[395] Sanclemente, G; De la Roche, CA; Escobar, CE, et al. Pentoxyfylline in toxic epidermal necrolysis and Stevens-Johnson syndrome. *Int J Dermatol* 1999; 38: 878-879.
[396] Frangogiannis, NG; Boridy, I; Mazhar, M, et al. Cyclophosphamide in the treatment of toxic epidermal necrolysis. *South Med J* 1996; 89: 1001-1003.
[397] Ang, CC; Tay, YK. Hematological abnormalities and the use of granulocyte-colony-stimulating factor in patients with Stevens-Johnson syndrome and toxic epidermal necrolysis. *Int J Dermatol* 2011; 50: 1570-1578.
[398] Inamo, Y; Okubo, T; Wada, M, et al. Intravenous ulinastatin therapy for Stevens-Johnson syndrome and toxic epidermal necrolysis in pediatric patients. Three case reports. *Int Arch Allergy Immunol* 2002; 127: 89-94.
[399] Egan, CA; Grant, WJ; Morris, SE, et al. Plasmapheresis as an adjunct treatment in toxic epidermal necrolysis. *J Am Acad Dermatol* 1999; 40: 458-461.
[400] Yamada, H; Takamori, K. Status of plasmapheresis for the treatment of toxic epidermal necrolysis in Japan. *Ther Apher Dial* 2008; 12: 355-359.
[401] Narita, YM; Hirahara, K; Mizukawa, Y, et al. Efficacy of plasmapheresis for the treatment of severe toxic epidermal necrolysis: Is cytokine expression analysis useful in predicting its therapeutic efficacy? *J Dermatol* 2011; 38: 236-245.

[402] Nomura, T; Abe, R; Fujimoto, K, et al. Plasma exchange; a promising treatment for toxic epidermal necrolysis with AIDS. *AIDS* 2004; 18: 2446-2448.

[403] Lissia, M; Figus, A; Rubino, C. Intravenous immunoglobulins and plasmapheresis combined treatment in patients with severe toxic epidermal necrolysis: preliminary report. *Br J Plast Surg* 2005; 58: 504-510.

[404] De Vriese, AS; Colardyn, FA; Philippe, JJ, et al. Cytokine removal during continuous hemofiltration in septic patients. *J Am Soc Nephrol* 1999; 10: 846-853.

[405] Furubacke, A; Berlin, G; Anderson, C, et al. Lack of significant treatment effect of plasma exchange in the treatment of drug-induced toxic epidermal necrolysis? *Intensive Care Med* 1999; 25: 1307-1310.

[406] Kumar, R; Dohlman, CH; Chodosh, J. Oral acetazolamide after Boston keratoprosthesis in Stevens-Johnson syndrome. *BMC Res Notes* 2012; 5: 205.

Index

B

C

D

E

H

I

K

L

M

N

O

P

R

S

T

U

V

W

X